SKELETAL RENEWAL
AND METABOLIC
BONE DISEASE

NEW ENGLAND JOURNAL OF MEDICINE

MEDICAL PROGRESS SERIES

SKELETAL RENEWAL AND METABOLIC BONE DISEASE

WILLIAM HAMILTON HARRIS, M.D.

ASSOCIATE CLINICAL PROFESSOR OF ORTHOPEDIC SURGERY,
HARVARD MEDICAL SCHOOL; VISITING ORTHOPEDIC SURGEON,
MASSACHUSETTS GENERAL HOSPITAL, BOSTON

ROBERT PROULX HEANEY, M.D.

PROFESSOR AND CHAIRMAN, DEPARTMENT OF MEDICINE,
CREIGHTON UNIVERSITY SCHOOL OF MEDICINE; DIRECTOR,
DEPARTMENT OF INTERNAL MEDICINE, CREIGHTON MEMORIAL
ST. JOSEPH HOSPITAL, OMAHA

LITTLE, BROWN AND COMPANY

BOSTON

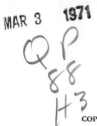

LIBRARY OF CONGRESS CATALOG CARD NO. 70-101759

FIRST EDITION

THIS MONOGRAPH FIRST APPEARED AS A MEDICAL PROGRESS REPORT IN THE NEW ENGLAND JOURNAL OF MEDICINE.

Published in Great Britain
by J. & A. Churchill Ltd., London

British Standard Book No. 7000 0172 7

PRINTED IN THE UNITED STATES OF AMERICA

To NAN AND BARBARA

PREFACE

THIS book is an attempt both to summarize existing knowledge of skeletal renewal and of the forces affecting and controlling it and to weave this information into a coherent fabric. The knowledge is largely the work of others; for the fabric we take responsibility. The field is so broad and so explicitly multidisciplinary that our treatment of it can only be accounted superficial by serious scientists working in any of its branches. We offer them our apologies. But this book has been written primarily for clinicians, for endocrinologists, internists and orthopedic surgeons, for students in these fields, and for clinical investigators attempting for the first time to study skeletal renewal. We hope it provides them a comprehensive overview of this fascinating field.

There are few areas of study today that have not been the subject of a knowledge explosion. Bone and calcium metabolism would certainly not be among those few. But the origins of this explosion are not always as obvious as they might seem. Certain of the investigative technics employed and many of the apparent breakthroughs in this field had been clearly worked out decades ago, only to be lost sight of. Intravital staining with tetracycline antibiotics, which has played such a key role in quantitative measurement of bone remodeling processes, was explicitly foreshadowed by the observation of Belchier in 1736 that madder root stains bones red. Similarly, by 1902 the broad outline of the relationships between osteoporosis, rickets, calcium deficiency and some as yet unknown factor (vitamin D had not yet been discovered) had been elucidated by at least two groups of German pathologists. Not only was such knowledge unused, it was lost; and the scientific community has only recently rediscovered facts which, in retrospect, had been clearly established many years ago.

But even if we admit that the origins of our present knowledge reach farther into the past than had been thought, it seems easy to discern the primary stimulus for the current growth phase; namely, the advent of nuclear weapons. The threat of bone-seeking fallout products created an urgent need to know more about the biology of bone and the mechanisms whereby mineral salts are stored in and released from its structure. At the same time, nuclear technology made isotopes readily available to biologic workers and thus handed them the tools needed to attack the problems it had created. The need and the tools alone might not have been enough, but happily both fell upon soil made fertile by such men as Albright, McLean, Howard, Armstrong and Schorr, to mention only a few of the giants who had prepared the way for this knowledge explosion. These men have been the teachers, advisers, beacons and inspiration of the authors, and we are pleased to acknowledge our great indebtedness, both personal and scientific, to them and to the work they accomplished which has made possible this attempt to synthesize current knowledge of skeletal renewal.

This work has been supported in part by grants from

the National Institute of Arthritis and Metabolic Diseases (AM-06375 and AM-07912), the National Institutes of Health, Public Health Service, United States Department of Health, Education, and Welfare.

W. H. H.
R. P. H.

CONTENTS

INTRODUCTION

THE skeleton, containing 99 per cent of the total body calcium, serves two major functions. First of all, it plays an important part in calcium homeostasis, both responding to and contributing to changes in calcium metabolism. Second, the structural integrity of the skeleton is essential for normal existence. Fractures, by far the most important abnormality of the skeletal system, occur with increasing frequency in the elderly because of decreasing strength of the skeleton. This weakness is due largely to a reduction in skeletal mass caused by an imbalance between the formation and the resorption of bone. Throughout life, even after cessation of longitudinal growth, cancellous and cortical bone are constantly being replaced by resorption of existing areas and by production of new deposits in microscopic amounts at many sites heterogeneously distributed throughout the skeleton. Changes in this balance between formation and resorption play a critical role in calcium homeostasis and underlie every disease that notably influences the adult skeleton.

In this review, in addition to summarizing current concepts of skeletal renewal, we will also look critically at the principal methods for studying skeletal remodeling and evaluate present knowledge of the more important metabolic bone diseases in this context. Although it is evident that remodeling is also essential for skeletal growth and development, we will confine our attention to the simpler situations afforded by remodeling in the mature skeleton. No attempt will be made to discuss the diseases in detail; they will be considered only in reference to abnormalities in skeletal renewal. Paget's disease will not be included. For a discussion of this subject, the reader is referred to the comprehensive article by Nagant de Deuxchaisnes and Krane.[1]

SKELETAL RENEWAL
AND METABOLIC
BONE DISEASE

1

MECHANISMS OF SKELETAL RENEWAL

Tissue Perspective

UNLIKE predominantly cellular tissues, in which renewal takes place largely at the molecular level, renewal of bone occurs at the tissue level. Whole volumes of bone are removed and replaced (Fig. 1). Not only is tissue replaced, but its architecture is altered as well. Resorption is produced either by osteoclastic "cutting cones," which tunnel through bone creating cavities approximately 200 microns (μ) in diameter and up to several millimeters in length, or by osteoclastic enlargement of existing vascular channels. The resulting cavities are filled in centripetally by osteoblasts depositing successive layers of highly oriented collagen fibers, which are subsequently mineralized. In cortical bone, for example, the primary circumferential lamellae are gradually replaced by longitudinally oriented, cylindrical structures termed Haversian systems, or osteons.[3] Thus, the size, shape and location of an osteon are determined by the resorption process.

Such remodeling continues throughout life, producing successive generations of osteons, partial resorption of circumferential lamellae and of preexisting osteons

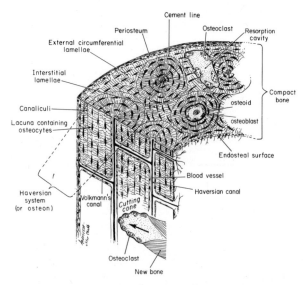

FIGURE 1. Three-dimensional diagram showing both a cross-section and a longitudinal section of the structure of the cortex of the shaft of a long bone. (Redrawn from Ham[1a] and from Johnson.[2])

leaving remnants termed *interstitial lamellae.* These may or may not retain their blood supply, depending on whether the resorption process proceeds across the previous osteon canal. If the blood supply is lost, the osteocytes that cannot be sustained by the diffusion of nutrition through canaliculi, an extensive network of protoplasmic extensions lying in minute bony channels, will die. Inevitably, older bone contains more such dead regions than young bone.[4]

These remodeling activities require continuous differentiation of specialized cells from the bone mesenchyme.[5] Indeed, all remodeling, even the resorption produced by osteolytic bone metastases, is mediated via the bone mesenchyme.

2

Cellular Basis for Remodeling

The three characteristic cell types of bone are the *osteoblast,* responsible both for matrix deposition and for its subsequent mineralization, the *osteocyte,* locked in its bony chamber and communicating with adjacent cells, and with vascular surfaces by means of canaliculi, and the *osteoclast* responsible for the virtually simultaneous dissolution and removal of matrix and mineral. The term *osteoclast* is here used more functionally than anatomically, for although one usually thinks of an osteoclast as a multinucleated giant cell, there is little doubt that clastic function is also mediated by certain mononuclear cells.

These cell types can be thought of as functional states of the bone mesenchyme: The osteoblast and the osteoclast particularly have a discrete existence only in relation to their functional activity. These specialized cell types must be produced by differentiation from mesenchymal precursors, and it seems likely that for most such cells this differentiation is irreversible. The cells do their job for a time, degenerate and are replaced by further mesenchymal induction. The life-span of the osteoclast appears to be from a few hours to at most a few days, and that of the osteoblast a few days to at most a few weeks of *effective* functional activity.[2] The actual life of osteoblasts may sometimes be longer than this because of long periods of functional arrest.

Bone Formation

In forming new bone, osteoblasts secrete soluble collagen, usually against a preexisting calcified surface.

This collagen aggregates extracellularly into an array of fibrils that in rapidly deposited bone has a feltlike, random orientation and in more slowly formed lamellar bone, a highly ordered, regular pattern. These collagen fibrils comprise 95 per cent of the organic matter of bone matrix, the other 5 per cent consisting of poorly characterized protein polysaccharides, glycoproteins and phospholipids. Altogether, these components occupy about 50 per cent of the volume of the matrix, the remainder being extracellular fluid. The electrolyte composition of this fluid is uncertain because osteoblasts may form a continuous membrane covering the surface on which they are working. Furthermore, there is some evidence that they actively transport materials across this membrane:[6] hence, they may well modify in an important way the small volume of extracellular fluid that they enclose.

As they work, osteoblasts elaborate matrix at a linear rate of approximately $1.0\,\mu$ per day, and the unmineralized matrix constitutes an osteoid "seam" or "border." Normally, these borders average 6 to $10\,\mu$ in thickness. Deep to this, at the "calcification front," there is an abrupt transition to matrix that is mineralized to 70 per cent of its ultimate full mineral capacity.[7] The width of these seams implies a lag of 5 to 10 days between matrix deposition and its subsequent mineralization, and indicates that the superficial layers of matrix are not capable of initiating or holding mineral deposits. This is also evident in the fact that mineral ions must pass through these superficial layers to reach the deeper calcification zone. Equally clear is the fact that this initially unmineralizable matrix must "mature" to calcify.

This maturation, under the control of the osteoblast,

proceeds in a sequence of histochemically recognizable zones involving changes in protein polysaccharides, phospholipids, phosphate enzymes (alkaline phosphatase, pyrophosphatase) and accumulation of metal ion, particularly zinc.[8] These changes attest to the extensive biochemical activity preceding initial mineral deposition, but the exact chemistry of that activity is obscure. The observation of lipid-staining materials at the calcification front[9] is of considerable interest, for this staining is absent in all osteomalacias regardless of cause, is restored by appropriate treatment and returns before mineralization. The material concerned appears to be a phospholipid, a finding that correlates with the well-known excretion of excess phosphoethanolamine (the nonlipid moiety of the cephalin molecule) by patients with hypophosphatasia, in which the essential bony lesion appears to be an enzymatic deficiency of matrix maturation.

A suitable nucleating configuration is somehow established, apparently within internal voids in the collagen fibril, presumably in association with phosphate binding by the collagen molecule.[10] Once nuclei reach a certain critical size, further mineralization proceeds spontaneously in the presence of normal calcium and phosphorus concentrations. A large share of the initially deposited mineral is crystallographically amorphous but exhibits a Ca:P molar ratio compatible with hydroxyapatite. In adult vertebrate bone this ratio usually is higher than the predicted value of 2:3 despite convincing evidence that some of the calcium lattice positions are unfilled (i.e., "defect" apatite). This paradox is best explained by the presence of carbonate, which in animals such as the turtle accounts for 13 per cent of total ash content.[10a] Carbonate content rises as the bone matures and is associated, at least temporally, with the conversion from a crystallographically amorphous configuration to the apatitic pattern characteristic of bone mineral. There is disagreement concerning the nature of bone carbonate, but current evidence is compatible with two distinct phases: an apatitic complex containing carbonate in the crystal lattice, and a separate $CaCO_3$ phase. Biltz and Pellegrino[10b] estimate that about half of bone carbonate in man exists as a separate phase, and that it is this function which is depleted in uremia and acidosis.

Extracellular fluid is roughly twice saturated with respect to hydroxyapatite. Hydroxyapatite is the crystal form of the majority of the calcium-phosphate deposits in bone. The initial calcium-phosphate solid phase is amorphous, but with time these amorphous deposits transform into hydroxyapatite. This complex subject is fully presented by Glimcher and Krane.[10] Hence, in the presence of suitable crystal nuclei, extracellular fluid will support crystal growth indefinitely (or until growth is limited by the available space or by poisoning of the crystal surface by adsorbed contaminants). On the other hand, hydroxyapatite nuclei do not spontaneously form in extracellular fluid under physiologic conditions. Therefore, extracellular fluid is termed "metastable"—that is, it is at one and the same time indefinitely stable in the absence of suitable nuclei and yet richly supports mineralization in the presence of suitable nuclei.[11, 12]

As the hydroxyapatite crystal forms *in situ,* it adsorbs onto its surface many of the substances present in the plasma ultrafiltrate. For the most part these are simply adventitious contaminants trapped in bone during its mineralization and have little direct significance either for the bone or for the body economy. However, inorganic pyrophosphate, normally present in plasma ultra-filtrates at concentrations in the range of 1 to 4 micrograms (μg) per liter, may be concentrated on the bone crystal surfaces and could alter the physical and chemical characteristics of the mineral. Hydroxyapatite crystals are known to adsorb large amounts of pyrophosphate from solutions with physiologic pyrophosphate concentration, and "coating" of such crystals both inhibits crystal growth or nucleation in supersaturated solutions and retards their dissolution in calcium-phosphate-free solutions.[12a] Bone is known to contain pyrophosphate, and pyrophosphate and hydroxyproline excretion rise proportionately under conditions of increased bone resorption.[12b]

Pyrophosphate is produced by a variety of intracellular reactions, particularly activation processes in which synthetic building blocks are coupled to nucleotides. Hence, pyrophosphate is provided not only by the blood but also by the cells covering the bone surface. Furthermore, the hydrolysis of pyrophosphate to orthophosphate by pyrophosphatases is almost certainly within the competence of the bone cells, and at least some of what is measured as alkaline phosphatase in the plasma or by histochemical technics is in fact a pyrophosphatase.[12c] These findings imply a crucial role for pyrophosphate at the interface between bone mineral and body fluids.

Pyrophosphate, present in only very small concentrations, affords the bone cells a means of controlling the reactivity of the canalicular and lacunar surface, and may be involved as well in that portion of nucleation and crystal growth under osteocytic control.

There is some evidence that osteoblasts may hasten nucleation by pumping calcium into the matrix,[6] but

7

such active pumping is probably not essential since nucleated matrixes (such as rachitic cartilage) will mineralize *in vitro* at usual calcium and phosphorus concentrations. In any event, the actively mineralizing matrix constitutes a kind of mineral trap and creates a mineral debt to which the organism must adjust. Mineral movement into new bone is initially rapid, and in compact cortical bone is known to reach 70 per cent of full mineralization within a few hours after matrix nucleation. This mineral deposition involves replacement of the water that originally occupied 50 per cent of the matrix volume. As water is displaced, further mineral diffusion is impeded, and the final 30 per cent of mineralization occurs slowly over a period of many weeks, usually 6 to 12. The initial rapid phase of mineralization is temporally and spatially related to osteoblast activity and has been termed *primary mineralization,* whereas the slower phase, termed *secondary mineralization,*[7] is independent of and frequently dissociated from the osteoblasts that initiated the process.

Although apparently distinct chemical processes, matrix formation and its subsequent maturation are coupled within the osteoblast, and a change in the rate of one of these functions is usually accompanied by a corresponding change in the other. Thus, it is common to find "resting osteoid"[13] borders of essentially normal width, as if both new matrix deposition and nucleation were stopped simultaneously. Even in the osteomalacias, in which osteoid borders may increase in width, sometimes greatly, the two activities appear to proceed at *almost* the same rate, though the time lag between deposition and mineralization may be increased several fold. The mechanisms of this remarkably tight coupling are entirely unknown.

Bone Resorption

The mechanisms of bone resorption are less well worked out. Osteoclastic cells appear to secrete enzymes onto the bone surface, and dissolve the mineral and digest the matrix at virtually the same moment. In the presence of parathyroid hormone (PTH), increased oxygen tension promotes resorption in organ culture;[14, 15] presumably, oxygen is necessary for the relatively huge amount of metabolic work involved in resorption. The process is associated with locally augmented blood flow and is known to involve acid production. The pH at resorbing sites has been shown to be lower than on other bone vascular surfaces,[15a] despite the fact that apatite solubilization consumes H^+.

Resorption appears to be a more rapid process than formation; however, linear resorption rate is difficult to measure under most circumstances. Johnson[2] has estimated that "cutting cones" advance at rates from 100 to 400 μ per day, but this rate may be much greater than that of other resorptive processes. Not only do they work more rapidly, but an osteoclast, during its brief life of, at most, a few days, resorbs six to eight times the volume of bone deposited by a single osteoblast through the whole of its life-span of several weeks.[8] Osteoclasts must operate from a free surface (vascular channel or trabecular, periosteal or endosteal surface), and in eroding bone they are usually no respecter of the age of the material through which they pass. The major exception seems to be an inability to resorb a surface covered with osteoid, though in organ culture even this is known to occur.[16] Normally, this would present no problem, for such surfaces are covered by osteoblasts, not clasts, but in the various osteomalacias,

80 per cent or more of all free surfaces may be covered with osteoid seams. Under such circumstances, osteoclastic function and the already compromised calcium-ion homeostasis become severely deranged.

Osteocyte Function

The capacity of osteocytes to resorb perilacunar bone[17] is most readily seen in situations associated with increased bone resorption, such as high levels of parathyroid activity[18] or vitamin A intoxication. However, the capacity is evident to a lesser extent in response to normal homeostatic stimuli as well.

It must be assumed that osteocytes can redeposit bone as well. This is inferred from the fact that enlarged lacunae have been seen only during times of forced bone resorption, and not after the stimulus to resorption has been terminated. This is highly circumstantial evidence, and to date a properly controlled experiment designed to establish osteocyte redeposition has not been done. However, lacunae in young bone are larger than those present after the bone ages, and hence, at least initially, osteocytes must possess osteoblastic competence. Finally, tetracycline deposits are frequently seen around some, but not all, osteocytes, suggesting new bone deposition at such sites.

Of the more than 1200 square meters of anatomic surface within the skeleton, 99 per cent is accounted for by the lacunar and canalicular surfaces.[2] Whereas this surface and its associated cellular activity have obvious implications for calcium homeostasis, they must be considered to have equally profound consequences for the mechanical properties of bony material itself. No volume of this extracellular material is more than a few microns from a cell-dominated surface, and periodic resorption and deposition would provide a means for surface renewal without the architectural changes associated with osteoblastic and osteoclastic function. All composite materials, such as the mineral-matrix composite of bone, change in their physical properties with time, but it is not yet known whether the properties of the bone material change sufficiently to have biologic consequence. To the extent that such a change did occur, one of the functions of the osteocyte would be the physical maintenance of the structural material within its domain.

2

METHODS OF STUDY OF IN VIVO
RATES OF SKELETAL RENEWAL

Calcium-Kinetic Methods

THE application of tracer technics for the study of bone mineral metabolism has been based on three important observations:

Over a period of several hours to several days, an intravenous calcium tracer mixes with less than 1 per cent of total body calcium.

Autoradiographs of bone demonstrate that newly formed areas of bone incorporate tracer and retain most of it as "hot spots" for the duration of the life-span of these areas.

Body tracer retention is considerably higher than can be accounted for by that contained within the miscible calcium pool; or equivalently, turnover of pool calcium is considerably greater than can be accounted for by excretion.

These observations mean simply that the vast bulk of skeletal calcium is exterior to the pool, that mineralization of new bone will remove calcium from the pool and that this process will ordinarily have a large enough effect on retention (or turnover) to be measurable.

There have been two principal approaches made to the analysis of tracer-kinetic data, and although the two can easily be shown to be mathematically equivalent, they differ in the type of observational data they employ and the point of view that they take toward the dynamics of body calcium. The first method is the formulation put forward by Bauer, Carlsson and Lindquist[19] to the effect that tracer retention is composed of two moieties: the portion contained within the exchangeable calcium pool and the portion that has been sequestered (removed from the pool) by mineralization of newly deposited bone matrix. Expressed mathematically this becomes

$$R(t) = E \cdot x(t) + A \int_0^t x(t) \, dt \qquad \text{(equation 1)}$$

where R is retention, E is the size of the exchangeable pool, A is the bone mineralization rate and x (t) is the plasma calcium specific activity. The focus of attention with this approach is tracer content of the body (or of any subregion, such as an isolated bone or bone specimen) and is most logically applicable where this quantity is directly measurable, as in studies with whole-body counters or when the tracer content of a bone sample is directly analyzed. The term for exchangeable calcium in this simple form of the equation assumes a uniform specific activity throughout the pool. Since this is known not to be the case (as described below), this equation is not well suited for accurate measurement of pool size. On the other hand, because the plasma integral can easily be obtained from a complete urine collection over the period of study or, as in rodents, from analysis of the tracer content of an incisor tooth, this method is especially valuable in situations in which adequate access to the plasma activity is limited.

The other major approach, proposed simultaneously by Heaney and Whedon[20] and by Aubert and Milhaud,[21] looks not so much at the tracer as at the behavior of the miscible pool, and employs the tracer primarily to measure pool size and turnover. This formulation states that pool turnover is adequately accounted for by excretion and bone mineralization on the output side, and by dietary calcium absorption and bone resorption on the input side. Thus:

$$
\text{Pool turnover} = \left\{
\begin{array}{l}
\begin{array}{l}\text{Calcium} \\ \text{accretion by} \\ \text{the skeleton}\end{array} + \begin{array}{l}\text{Urine} \\ \text{calcium}\end{array} + \begin{array}{l}\text{Endogenous} \\ \text{fecal} \\ \text{calcium}\end{array} \\
\\
\begin{array}{l}\text{Dietary} \\ \text{calcium} \\ \text{absorption}\end{array} + \begin{array}{l}\text{Calcium} \\ \text{removed from} \\ \text{the skeleton}\end{array}
\end{array}
\right.
\qquad \text{(equation 2)}
$$

This approach, although mathematically equivalent to the Bauer-Carlsson-Lindquist formulation, is empirically best suited to situations in which pool specific activity is directly measurable and in which actual isotope retention is not. It has the further advantage of making explicit provision for bone resorption, which the Bauer-Carlsson-Lindquist formulation cannot do, and is more easily adapted to handling the problem of nonuniform specific activity in the various pool compartments.

In both formulations, tracer retention in bone is determined by (and hence can be used to measure) the aggregate of several different activities, as follows:

$$
\begin{array}{l}\text{Tracer} \\ \text{uptake} \\ \text{(accretion)}\end{array} \left\{
\begin{array}{l}
\left.\begin{array}{l}\text{Primary mineralization} \\ \text{Secondary mineralization} \\ \text{Periosteocytic ``deposition''}\end{array}\right\} \text{Bone mineralization} \\
\\
\text{Long-term exchange}
\end{array}
\right.
$$

Only primary mineralization is closely associated with osteoblastic activity, and even here there is a lag of 6 to 10 days between matrix deposition and its subsequent mineralization. An important consequence of the delay

15

is the fact that diseases or treatments that alter osteoblast activity will not be fully reflected immediately in their effect on calcium tracer uptake by bone. It is probable that a minimum of several weeks is required after such a change in osteoblast activity before mineral-based measurements accurately reflect matrix deposition.

However, primary and secondary mineralization and periosteocytic deposition all represent *net* calcium accumulation in bone, and in the presence of a normal stoichiometric relation of mineral to matrix, they represent as valid a measure of bone formation as would direct measurement of matrix deposition. And in fact, because they include the periosteocytic deposition (to whatever extent it occurs), these mineral uptake phenomena are a more complete measure of total bone formation than can ordinarily be provided by the microscopical methods. For the same reason, the kinetic measurement of resorption represents the sum of mineral released by osteoclastic resorption and periosteocytic osteolysis.

The phrase *long-term exchange* refers to the fact that preformed bone mineral is not completely isolated from body-fluid calcium, but instead exchanges with it very slowly, although at a rate so low in man that equilibrium would take longer than a human life-span. This exchange, of course, does not involve net transfer of calcium in either direction, but before equilibrium, much more tracer will move into the diffuse component of bone than comes out, and this difference will be seen by the kinetic methods as if it represented net mineral transport. This fact makes the accretion value somewhat higher than the true value for net bone mineralization (bone formation). Similarly, the contrary exchange of unlabeled calcium out of the diffuse component makes the kinetic resorption value higher than the actual net removal of mineral from bone.

In smaller animals, this long-term exchange process replaces 10 to 20 per cent of the total skeletal calcium per year.[22] Adequate, comparable data for normal adult man are not available, but preliminary data from terminal patients suggest a rate in the range of 1 to 2 per cent per year.[23] This may not be representative, but, if applicable, would amount to between 8 and 15 per cent of the normal accretion and resorption values (as indicated later).

Even if negligible under normal conditions, long-term exchange might appreciably influence accretion and mineral removal measurements in disease. The contact between preformed mineral and the body fluid takes place on the free surfaces of bone. These include lacunar and canalicular surfaces as well as the more obvious surface areas of cortical and trabecular bone, and amount to more than 1200 square meters, 99 per cent of which is osteocytic. Virtually all this surface is dominated by bone cells, and it must be assumed that these cells moderate the underlying physiochemical processes of simple exchange. We have already commented on the possible role of ions such as pyrophosphate in these surface interactions.

Actually, this presents the problem of long-term exchange in its worst possible light. Exchange involving only the superficial 1-μ layer of this osteocyte and canalicular surface is sufficient to account for the total isotope of the diffuse component. However, by the same token, actual bone resorption and deposition on this surface would suffice just as well, and as we have remarked earlier, it is probable that such resorption and deposition do normally occur on certain of these surfaces. Unfortunately, whereas this activity can be detected by morphologic methods, it cannot be measured by them; there is no independent method for calibrating all aspects of the mineral kinetic measurements.

Specific activity, the basic measurement of the kinetic methods, is a reflection of tracer *concentration,* not of content, within a system. Although excretion and accretion are commonly thought to be responsible for decline in specific activity because they remove tracer from the pool, technically they are not. Rather, it is the entrance of unlabeled calcium into the pool that is responsible for the fall in specific activity. Gastrointestinal absorption and return of calcium from bone are the two routes of entry of this unlabeled calcium into the pool.

Thus, since the turnover-difference method is based on pool specific activity, if it measures anything at all, it measures calcium release from bone first and most directly, whereas the Bauer-Carlsson-Lindquist equation, based on system content, more directly measures the effects of accretion.

The various exchangeable calcium compartments can be accurately thought of only as a great number of small units exchanging more or less directly with plasma calcium and with a continuous distribution of exchange rates, from very rapid to very slow. Fortunately, for purposes of analysis this distribution appears to fall into three major groups: those mixing very rapidly with plasma and coming into equilibrium in 20 minutes or less after intravenous injection; a much slower intermediate group requiring two to three days to equilibrate with plasma; and finally a whole series of very much slower units composed almost exclusively of the diffuse component of bone.* The last is ignored in most attempts at pool analysis, and as we have seen, enters into kinetic calculations only because it falsely elevates formation and resorption values. The first two groups can be reasonably well approximated by two compartments and are the basis for the now commonly employed two-compartment model.[25] The rapid compartment consists of plasma calcium, most or all of the extracellular-fluid calcium, a very thin layer of surface calcium in bone, particularly along vascular channels, and an indeterminate fraction of cellular calcium. The slower compartment consists of a part of the cellular calcium, calcium in avascular tissues such as cartilage, fibrous tissue, dystrophic or metastatic calcium deposits, and probably also a more remote portion of bone calcium.

In the two-compartment model, the system is conceived as giving calcium to and receiving it from a third, infinitely large compartment, which represents both calcium outside the organism and the bulk of skeletal calcium. These processes, designated as "turnover," can be evaluated most easily by direct graphic analysis of the plasma specific-activity curve, expressed as a two-term exponential equation, as in Figure 2.†

---

* Elaborate multicompartmental analysis (such as that of Neer et al.[24]) requiring extensive computer facilities can break these groups down still further and can draw into the scheme some of the more rapid components of long-term exchange as well. These technics, though theoretically preferable, are not widely applicable and have not appeared as yet to add to the information provided by the simpler two-compartment model.

† As indicated in Figure 2, the constants employed in equation 3 represent the slopes and y-intercepts of the two straight lines into which the curve can be graphically decomposed. Neither these constants nor the separate terms of equation 3 bear any simple relation to the individual compartments of the model. The review by Heaney[25] and the treatise by A. K. Solomon[25a] present the derivation of these

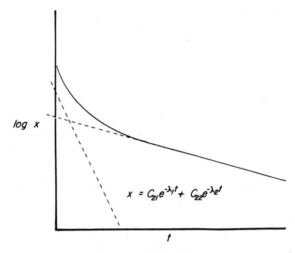

FIGURE 2. Plasma calcium specific-activity curve, expressed as a two-term exponential equation. The coefficients (C_{21} and C_{22}) represent the y-axis intercepts, and the exponents (λ_1 and λ_2), the slopes of the two straight lines into which the curve has been graphically decomposed.

$$\text{Turnover} = \frac{\lambda_2}{C_{22} + C_{21}\dfrac{\lambda_2}{\lambda_1}} \qquad \text{(equation 3)}$$

Given this value for turnover, solution of equation 2 for accretion and calcium removal from bone then requires only direct chemical measurement of urine calcium, calculation of endogenous fecal calcium by means of tracer clearance through the gastrointestinal tract or measurement of calcium absorption.[25, 26]

Application of this approach to available normal data, derived from a multilaboratory composite reference standard,[27] yields the following values for calcium:

---

equations and the mathematical relation of the constants to the compartments of the model.

Fast compartment	1.66 gm	Intercompart-mental flux	0.971 gm/day
Slow compartment	3.13 gm	External turn-over	0.617 gm/day
Total pool	4.79 gm	Accretion	0.346 gm/day

Proper interpretation of the calcium kinetic data depends upon an understanding not only of what the technics can do but also of what they cannot. The principal limitations of the methods can be summarized briefly: First of all, calcium tracers provide a measure of net mineral movement into bone. This is a valid index of bone formation, but it is not the same as a direct measure of osteoblast activity. Furthermore, in any disease in which there is a dissociation between mineral and matrix deposition, as in osteomalacia or rickets, the mineral kinetic methods may not be appropriate. Second, in intact human patients total-body calcium kinetic methods necessarily average the activity of the entire skeleton, and hence will be a poor tool for the study of essentially local bone disease. Third, extremely rapid bone turnover, as in Paget's disease, may return tracer-containing bone by way of resorption to the miscible pool before equilibrium has been achieved within that pool, and hence render quantitative kinetic analysis meaningless. Fourth, nonosseous calcific deposits may contribute to what is measured by accretion or calcium return from the skeleton. Although such deposits may amount to several grams of calcium in most elderly persons, there is little evidence that these deposits turn over rapidly enough to perturb kinetic analysis in such cases. However, in the uremic syndromes or in a variety of hypercalcemic diseases, in both of which changing metastatic calcification may occur, such changes will certainly be reflected in the kinetic analysis.

Morphometric Methods

The two types of quantitative microscopical technics used to assess rates of skeletal renewal are studies of surface activity and studies of volume changes using dual or multiple intravital labels.

Surface Measurements

The percentage of total bone surface, excluding periosteocytic and canalicular surfaces, occupied by formation has been determined with the use of several indexes, including the presence of osteoid seams,[28] a "hot spot" on autoradiography, tetracycline uptake[29] and the characteristic appearance of primary mineralization surfaces on microradiography.[30] Estimating new bone surface from osteoid seams is misleading because even in normal subjects not all the osteoid seams are being actively mineralized;[28] furthermore, the proportion of this "resting osteoid" increases with age, and in diseases such as osteomalacia a high disparity develops between the percentage of surface occupied by osteoid and the percentage of bone surface actually undergoing mineral growth.[31] Tetracycline uptake[32] and microradiography, since they both accurately identify *active* growing surfaces with high resolution, currently are widely used in formation studies. Resorption surfaces are identified by the scalloped appearance of the surface or by the presence of multinucleated osteoclasts.

Surface measurements are expressed as a fraction of the total morphologic bone surface in a given section in which evidence of resorbing or forming activity can be detected. Since all bone remodeling must proceed from a surface, these surface measurements are well suited to detect changes in remodeling activity; furthermore, they offer data directly relevant to both formation and resorption. Data from these technics first demonstrated the marked increase in resorption surface over formation surface in osteoporotic patients,[30, 33] the age-related increase in resorption surface compared to formation surface in elderly nonosteoporotic patients[30] and the increase in resorption surface in patients with hyperparathyroidism who did not have radiologic evidence of bone disease.[34] To understand surface-activity values it is necessary to bear in mind, however, that these values are fractional and not absolute, and that changes in total surface (for example, increased porosity) could alter the total amount of formation without any change in the *percentage* of surface involved.

If these surface measurements are to be interpreted in terms of *volumes* of bone formed or resorbed per unit time, three questions must be answered: Is the linear rate of activity at the surface constant—that is, is it the same as in normal subjects, and is it the same as at other times in this same patient? Is the activity present in that section at the instant of sacrifice truly representative of activity at that site over a long time? And is the activity found in the biopsy material from that site representative of the skeleton as a whole?

One can determine the linear rate of formation, called the appositional growth rate, by giving two tetracycline labels separated by a known interval and measuring the bone deposition occurring between the two markers. Although the appositional growth rate in cortical bone in dogs and man is generally about 1μ per day, important differences exist in young dogs from site to site,[35] decreases in rate exist between young and old dogs,[35] and in the rib of the adult human being the appositional growth rate decreases with age.[13] Osteomalacia dramatically reduces the appositional growth rate.[13, 31] Subtle changes that might exist in other pathologic states are beyond resolution by the dual marker method. The appositional growth rate, therefore, is subject to changes that can alter the net amount of formation, independently of changes in the amount of surface occupied by formation. The linear rate of bone resorption, as noted above, is much more difficult to measure. Furthermore, monocytic and osteocytic resorption is not measured by the usual technics, and some error is often introduced by the fact that resorption is usually too focal to extend fully throughout the thickness of a microscopical section.

Baylink and co-workers have shown that linear resorption rates rise as the plasma calcium falls, and that this rise is retarded by vitamin D deficiency.[35a] It seems likely that further work will reveal extensive modulation of the linear resorption rate under both disease conditions and pharmacologic intervention.

If the interval between the cessation of resorption and the initiation of formation (that is, the "turnaround time") were prolonged, the prevalence of areas of apparent resorption surface would exceed the true amount of active resorption surface. Wu, Jett and Frost[36] calculate that in the human rib the turn-around time increases with age. In experimental rickets Kelly[37] found many resorption cavities lined with osteoid. This is never seen normally and also indicates an increased turn-around time. Jowsey[38] reports that normally the microradiographic appearance of sites of inactive resorption can be identified and hence discounted.

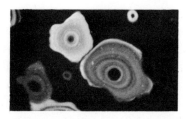

FIGURE 3. Fluorescent photomicrograph of a cross-section of canine tibia ($\times 100$), showing several osteons labeled in a color-coded, long-duration experiment. The daily administration of tetracycline identifies the volume of new bone formed during the entire duration of labeling. The use of two different tetracyclines in separate labeling periods permits identification of the growth in each period (see text). Intermittency of growth (which occurs normally), delays in mineralization such as occur in osteomalacia and changes in the appositional growth rate introduce no errors in this technic because only newly mineralized bone is counted and all newly mineralized bone is accurately identified by the tetracycline labels.

Volume Measurements

Dual or continuous intravital markers are employed to measure the volume of bone deposited between two defined points in time, and hence they yield formation *rates*. Markers such as the tetracyclines are preferentially localized in all bone-forming surfaces at the time they are in the circulating blood,[32] and they accurately identify such bone when undemineralized sections are examined under ultraviolet light (Fig. 3). Short-duration labels are frequently used to indicate the beginning and end of experimental periods, but will fail to provide a double label for bone formation that started after the first label, stopped before the second or was completed wholly within the interval between the labels. For this reason, continuous labeling during an entire experimental period is preferred. Different experimental periods can be clearly demarcated by the use of two tetracyclines with different color fluorescence[39] (Fig. 3).

Measurements of the bone deposited during the labeling period are expressed as a fraction of the total cross-sectional area. Volume measurements are referred to the total volume in the section examined and are usually extrapolated to an annual figure. These methods allow direct assessment of appositional growth rate and the volume of bone formed in a unit time, as well as comparison of two intervals in the same section, and provide graphic evidence of the heterogeneity of skeletal remodeling.

An example of these aspects of color-coded volume labeling is provided by a study in three adult dogs labeled daily for 12 weeks with oxytetracycline and subsequently each day for 12 weeks with demethyl-chlortetracycline. Since the fluorescent emission of the two tetracyclines in bone is distinctive, all growth dur-

TABLE 1. *Differences from Site to Site in the Rate of Skeletal Renewal within the Tibia in Three Normal Mature Dogs, as Indicated by Labeling with Two Tetracyclines*

| | Percentage of Existing Bone Replaced/Yr. | | | | | |
| | Dog 30 | | Dog 32 | | Dog 7 | |
Site	1st Period*	2nd Period*	1st Period*	2nd Period*	1st Period*	2nd Period*
Proximal metaphysis	12.0	2.8	11.4	15.0	11.8	7.0
Proximal diaphysis	8.7	1.4	14.3	13.2	9.0	7.5
Distal diaphysis	4.0	6.4	9.2	23.8	9.5	12.0
Distal metaphysis	7.3	4.0	12.9	26.7	5.7	12.9

* Each labeling period 84 days.

TABLE 2. *Annual Rate of Skeletal Renewal in Cortical Bone in Three Normal Mature Dogs**

Dog No.	Percentage of Existing Bone Replaced/Yr.	
	Long Bones	Ribs
30	4.7	14.0
32	11.2	44.0
7	9.5	18.5

* Adapted from Harris et al.[39]

ing each of the two three-month intervals was distinguishable. Table 1 shows a comparison of the rate of new bone formed, expressed for each 12-week interval as the percentage of the total bone present that would have been replaced annually, for four sites in the tibia of the three dogs. In Table 2 the average annual rate of formation for long bones is given for each dog, along with the annual average figure for ribs. Obviously, metabolic activity in the ribs differs markedly from that in long bones, and within long bones marked differences exist from site to site as well as from time to time at the same site. These figures, striking as they are, already contain a large averaging factor since each figure in Table 1 is the average of four sections from each skeletal site, and the total growth recorded occurred over an 84-day interval.

Such long-duration, color-coded tetracycline methods enable the use of individual subjects as their own control, a distinct advantage in view of the heterogeneity in formation rates.

A special problem of all microscopical studies is the marked decrease in accuracy of assessment of activity in cancellous bone. This is due to the facts that the trabeculae are usually much thinner than the section thickness itself, and that they are not oriented at right angles to the section. Thus, a large number of oblique surfaces, which are difficult or impossible to quantitate accurately, are encountered. This difficulty in dealing with cancellous bone is particularly important in view of the estimation that cancellous bone accounts for 50 per cent of the skeletal turnover, in spite of amounting to only one fifth of the total skeletal mass.[2]

In summary, the microscopical methods provide direct measurement of fractional formation and resorption surface, and of fractional formation volume. Because they involve direct assessment of skeletal tissue, they obviate some of the problems of the tracer-balance or turnover-difference technics. Pool size, errors in fecal losses and long-term exchange are not notable factors. However, to use microscopical technics, biopsies must be taken, and a large sample is necessary to overcome heterogeneity in skeletal metabolic activity unless marked changes are present. Furthermore, the accuracy of microscopical methods in cancellous bone is limited, and such procedures are inapplicable to periosteocytic remodeling.

Other Methods

Hydroxyproline

The measurement of daily urinary excretion of hydroxyproline, the unique amino acid found almost exclusively in collagen and not reused in the synthesis of new collagen, held promise of providing specific data on bone resorption. However, because of excretion of hydroxyproline from nonosseous sources of collagen and oxidation of hydroxyproline, as well as because of variable contributions to the total urinary hydroxyproline from increased synthesis rather than from resorption, it has been impossible to realize this expectation fully. Urinary hydroxyproline correlates fairly well with bone resorption in certain states, but also parallels serum alkaline phosphatase levels and measurements of increased bone formation in others. It seems to correlate best with periods of high skeletal turnover.[40] This is not too surprising since it receives contributions from both formation and resorption processes in bone. Radioactive hydroxyproline in the urine can be used more accurately to indicate bone resorption in animals given labeled proline weeks or months previously.[41]

Quantitative Radiography

Another major avenue of attack on problems of skeletal dynamics involves use of x-ray determination of such points as cortical thickness of long bones and relative density measurements of the lumbar spine in different populations or in the same population over time.[42, 43] The findings will be discussed in Chapter 4, but suffice it to say here that extensive radiographic studies of lumbar vertebrae, metacarpals, femurs and so forth have revealed a universal, progressive loss of skeletal mass in adults with age—data not apparent with any other technic. The development of photon-beam scan technics has made possible the assessment *in vivo* of subtle changes and has increased the ability to follow the effect of perturbations of skeletal metabolism.[44]

Calcium Balance

Balance data are required by the Bauer-Carlsson-Lindquist formula if calcium removal from the skeleton is to be estimated, and at a minimum, complete excreta collections are necessary for the turnover-difference methods. These technics are expensive and time-consuming, and have recently come under attack as being grossly inaccurate and misleading.[45] There is systematic error that tends to make balance measurement more positive than actual balance, but with care this error can be minimized. The use of chromic oxide or polyethylene glycol has improved timing of fecal collections, and at the same time corrects for the fraction of the systematic error caused by incomplete fecal collections.

Early studies with whole-body counters suggested that actual tracer retention was considerably less than could be explained by excretory losses, and it was concluded that the balance measurements were in error. They may have been in certain cases, but recent work employing both modern whole-body counters and careful balance procedures has produced essentially equivalent figures for isotope retention.[46, 46a] Rose[47] estimates current balance technics to be accurate to 10 per cent on a six-day period and to 3 per cent on duplicate six-day studies.

3

CONTROL OF SKELETAL
REMODELING

Control Mechanics

FROM the point of view of control mechanics, remodeling exhibits two control loops with negative feedback characteristics: parathyroid-calcitonin-mediated resorption, serving calcium homeostasis; and the effects of mechanical forces on the skeleton, whereby the mass and arrangement of the skeletal material is altered to meet changing structural needs. The first is essentially a systemic process and the second a local phenomenon, though the two importantly interact at the level of the cells that mediate them. In addition, a very large number of factors, including mineral nutrition, hormonal balance, systemic or local disease and aging, have important skeletal effects that interact with the control system.

Calcium homeostasis is mediated by parathyroid hormone and, at least in young animals, calcitonin. The skeletal effects of these hormones are exerted predominantly on the resorptive process. PTH stimulates mesenchymal proliferation and osteoclast induction, and accelerates the osteolytic activity of osteocytes. The initial calcium release from bone in response to PTH occurs too rapidly to be accounted for by cell modulation, and is believed to be due to osteocytic osteolysis. Some of this rapid phase may result from stimulation of existing osteoclasts as well. However, it appears that the principal effect of the hormone is a marked increase in the number of osteoclasts. Vitamin D seems to be required for the osseous effects of PTH, and when present in pharmacologic concentrations will stimulate both osteocytic and osteoclastic resorption. Calcitonin directly inhibits the resorptive process, and, although inhibition occurs in the absence of PTH, the effects are most obvious when there are high levels of resorption. Its rapidity of action indicates clearly that the resorptive process, and not osteoclast differentiation, is its major focus of action.

Osteoclastic proliferation is not necessarily equivalent to enhanced resorption. A number of factors are known to interfere with osteoclast function, and there are undoubtedly many more to be discovered. Vitamin D deficiency certainly reduces the efficiency of osteoclast work, and resorptive response to a constant level of PTH has more recently been found to vary inversely with the concentration of both calcium[48] and phosphorus[49] in the medium. These latter effects constitute a kind of end-product inhibition analogous to the many well-recognized biochemical examples of such intrinsic regulatory activity. Perhaps most significant is the fact that this reciprocal inhibition constitutes the only known control loop influencing the concentration of phosphate in extracellular fluid.

Heparin is known to enhance resorptive response to PTH in organ culture,[50] and fluoride to inhibit it,[51] though the fluoride effect leads to marked increases in osteoclast numbers, presumably because of increasing

PTH production in an attempt to offset the reduced efficiency of each osteoclast.[52] Similarly, the osteitis fibrosa of renal osteodystrophy and of some osteomalacias is frequently—if not invariably—more striking than the elevation of bone resorption, suggesting that *tissue* response to PTH is dissociated from *chemical-work* response to the hormone. The physiologic significance of these findings can be summarized in two ways: In the first place, PTH increases the osteoclast population and stimulates osteocytic osteolysis. It is not definitely known to alter the specific function of each osteoclast. Other things being equal, however, increased osteoclasts mean increased bone resorption. Second, osteoclast function may be enhanced or inhibited by a large variety of agencies acting at one or more sites distal to the effect of PTH, and these alterations may produce resorption rates considerably greater or less than the histologic pattern might suggest.

The controlling influence exerted by mechanical forces has been recognized for over 100 years and has been formulated as Wolff's law: Every change in the function of a bone is followed by certain definite changes in its internal architecture and its external conformation. Well-recognized examples include the fact that the triangular cross-section of the tibia is dependent on weight-bearing and muscular attachments, and that, in the young, a fibula used to bridge a tibial defect hypertrophies to approach the size of a normal tibia. Equally well known is the osteoporosis that develops as a result of immobilization or disuse.

Of the many theories proposed to explain how mechanical forces communicate with the cells responsible for bone formation and resorption, the most appealing has been the postulation of induced electrical fields mediating this information exchange.[53] Deformation of macroscopic units of bone produces a charge separation in the millivolt range, and current flow on the order of 10^{-15} amperes, both of which are proportional to the applied force. Many crystalline (or semicrystalline) materials—including both bone collagen and its associated mineral—exhibit piezoelectrical properties. In bone, regions under tension act as anode, and compressed regions as cathode. Currents of this magnitude have been shown to be capable of the spatial orientation of collagen fibrils as they aggregate from the solution phase, and are known to have definite effects on regeneration blastemas in amphibia.[54]

The negative-feedback characteristic of this mechanism lies in the fact that bone accumulates about the cathodal region of this system, reducing the compressive stress and hence reducing the electrical effects produced by an applied force. To the extent that this hypothesis applies to real bone remodeling, its most obvious example may well be the deposition of new bone on the concave (compressed) side of a long bone deformed because of rickets or a malaligned fracture. It is harder to visualize its application to the more usual situation in which tensile, compressive and shear forces must alternate rapidly and unpredictably within most bony regions, however small; remodeling takes place over extended periods, whereas mechanically induced electrical fields are ephemeral. Undoubtedly, certain field strengths and configurations predominate in different bony volumes, and a sort of averaging effect may suffice to determine local bone-remodeling activity.

The mechanisms by which the bone mesenchyme responds to mechanical stimuli (whether or not mediated by electrical signals) are uncertain. In general, heavy usage leads to heavy bones, but the cellular response is discouragingly complex. The sequence of changes after a major decrease in mechanical stresses will be described in Chapter 6 in the section Local Osteoporosis. For these purposes it is enough to note that the primary change produced by disuse is increased resorption; presumably, the opposite occurs with increased stress, but suitable experiments to test this hypothesis have not been done. Mechanical forces appear to have a slightly stimulating effect on formation as well, but in all the experiments performed to date, this action has been far less striking than the resorptive effects.

There are three important aspects of remodeling control: magnitude (or rate); location; and balance (between formation and resorption). PTH and mechanical forces influence the magnitude, and mechanical forces to some extent the location, but other important factors condition even these responses. Excess parathyroid secretion is characteristically expressed as subperiosteal resorption; disuse produces resorption first in the metaphysis and then endosteally.[55] Alterations in blood flow associated with these processes may make the decisive difference between the two resorption patterns, but obviously much more needs to be learned about such local factors.

Of great interest is the interaction between PTH and mechanical forces. The skeleton is continuously subjected both to the essentially uniform influence of PTH and to complex and changing mechanical forces. Parathyroidectomy markedly retards the development of disuse osteoporosis (whether from denervation or casting).[56, 57] These observations suggest not that this local change is systemically mediated, but that local mechanical factors modify the response of bone to systemic stimuli. In other words mechanically stressed bone is less sensitive to homeostatic forces than unused bone.

At the risk of building too complex a structure on a very small foundation, one can speculate that PTH (with calcitonin) is a major determinant of the magnitude of all remodeling, structural as well as homeostatic, and mechanical forces the major determinant of where that remodeling occurs. Certainly, skeletal turnover is markedly reduced in hypoparathyroidism, even though mechanical forces and all other endocrine factors remain unchanged.

Coupling of Resorption and Formation

One of the more striking, and probably unexpected, results to emerge from calcium kinetic studies has been the observation that bone formation and resorption tend to change in the same direction. Figure 4 presents values of bone accretion rate in over 100 studies performed in the laboratory of R. P. Heaney, plotted as a function of calcium release from bone, and demonstrates graphically the close coupling that exists between these two activities over two full orders of magnitude. The patients represented by this graph had a wide spectrum of diseases, from hyperparathyroidism, acromegaly and Paget's disease on the high end of the spectrum to hypoparathyroidism on the low end. In all of them, the level of calcium release was a reliable predictor of the level of accretion, and vice versa. The spread about the identity relation reflects the fact of positive and negative balance, but it is clear that the degree of disparity between formation and resorption (that is, the magnitude of balance) is far smaller than

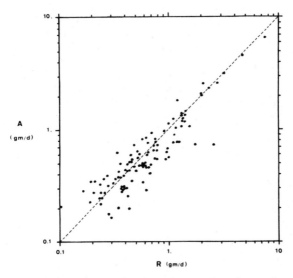

FIGURE 4. Calcium return (R) from bone, plotted as a function of calcium accretion (A) in 108 patients with a wide variety of disorders affecting calcium metabolism.

the magnitude of the component skeletal-turnover processes at all levels except the lower remodeling rates. Morphologic studies have shown this type of parallel change in formation and resorption surface in all disorders examined to date with the exception of Cushing's syndrome, in which Riggs, Jowsey and Kelly[58] have reported a decreased amount of formation surface and an increased amount of resorption surface.

Situations during which formation and resorption change in opposite directions undoubtedly occur, such as early in the development of disuse osteoporosis, but these appear to be transient and to be offset by more slowly acting mechanisms that couple formation to resorption. What can be said of these coupling mechanisms? Three possible explanations should be men-

37

tioned. The first is homeostatic and arises from the mineral debt created by nucleated bone matrix. This debt constitutes a part of the demand to which the parathyroid glands are continuously reacting, and since the level of PTH is one of the determinants of bone resorption, one can see immediately that high levels of bone formation will tend to produce high levels of resorption, for unless the calcium demands of increased formation can be met in some other way, such as by sudden changes in calcium intake from the diet, they will inevitably lead to increased PTH secretion and bone resorption. This mechanism acts systemically, involves the entire skeleton, is short lived and amounts to a situation in which prior formation determines subsequent resorption.

Another possible explanation of coupling is the mechanical force–piezoelectrical system discussed earlier. Local bone resorption, by reducing structural volume, concentrates applied forces in the remaining bone, and this necessarily leads to increased strain. Presumably, this would increase the stimulus for local bone repair. This scheme is essentially local, acts over a period of many months and amounts to a situation in which prior resorption determines subsequent formation. The third explanation consists of an analogous local mechanism proposed by Wu, Jett and Frost.[36] They have suggested that the induction of specialized bony cells from the mesenchyme proceeds in a predetermined sequence: first osteoclasts and then osteoblasts, so that, even on free surfaces, resorption always precedes formation. There is doubt whether this sequence does in fact always occur,[59] but the coupling itself seems incontrovertible, even if its mechanism is problematic.

4

AGE-RELATED CHANGES IN THE ADULT SKELETON

Quantitative Changes

BEGINNING about the fourth decade, the entire skeletal mass decreases with age, a most important observation. This statement is true of cancellous and cortical bone, appendicular as well as axial skeleton, both sexes and all races.[42] The only region that does not follow this pattern is the skull. Five significant features of this universal loss of skeletal mass are as follows: Among young adults, the skeletal mass is greater in males than females and greater in blacks than whites in America; the loss begins earlier in females than in males; the onset of loss in females antedates the menopause; loss in the female is distinctly accelerated after the menopause; and the rate of loss is faster in whites than in blacks.

Because the maximum skeletal mass at maturity is less for the white female than for the male or the Negro of either sex, and because the loss begins earlier in the female and proceeds at a more rapid rate after the menopause, net skeletal mass is lowest in the post-menopausal white female.

Resorption, particularly at endosteal surfaces, exceeds formation; hence, in the shafts of long bones, the characteristic change with age is cortical thinning. In certain regions, such as the midshaft of the femur, the two processes of periosteal deposition and endosteal resorption result in a progressive enlargement as well as thinning of the cortex.[60] Despite some decreases in mass, the increase in shaft diameter usually produces an increase in structural rigidity. An expanded shaft absorbs less stress and transfers more of it to the intertrochanteric and femoral-neck regions, which are already weakened by the age-related loss of skeletal mass.

Differences in the rate of loss of cortical thickness exist throughout the skeleton, but such losses clearly affect weight-bearing as well as non-weight-bearing bones. Regional differences may exist within a single bone. For example, areas of the femoral cortex that are of smaller volume at skeletal maturity are preferentially subject to progressive loss with age, whereas regions that were larger at maturity remain almost untouched by the age-related losses.[61] Taller patients of both sexes lose less rapidly because of more rapid periosteal new bone formation. Since they have a larger skeleton at full skeletal maturity, their skeletal mass remains high even at advanced age as compared to that of smaller persons.

Qualitative Changes

In addition to the changes in mass occurring with age throughout the skeleton, qualitative changes occur.[4, 62] An increasing number of osteons remain incompletely closed despite a decrease in the total number of newly formed osteons. This indicates an aberration in the normal process of completion of the formation of osteons. The time lag between the cessation of resorption at a resorption cavity and the initiation of formation within that cavity increases with age.[63] Moreover, an increasing number of osteons are less completely mineralized. Either they failed to complete their secondary mineralization or they are subject to a form of unusual mineral loss.[4]

The other important finding occurring with age is the increase in nonviable segments in cortical bone. Plugging of osteon canals, osteocyte death, osteocyte lacunae hypermineralization, and hypermineralization of interstitial lamellar segments may all be evidence of a progressive increase in regional avascularity in cortical bone with age.[4, 62] However, Newton-John and Morgan[64] calculate that the frequency of fracture parallels the frequency of people with reduced mineral mass, and believe that no qualitative change is necessary to explain the data. Studies of the physical properties of vertebrae support this opinion.[65]

5

THE ROLE OF HORMONES IN
SKELETAL RENEWAL

Calcitonin

ONE of the most exciting areas of advance in understanding skeletal physiology during the past seven years has been the discovery and study of calcitonin, a single-chain polypeptide hormone of 32 amino acids[66] and a molecular weight of about 3600, that is produced by the ultimobranchial body in lower forms and by the "C" cells of the thyroid gland (derived from the ultimobranchial tissue) in man. The recent review by Foster[67] and the publication of recent symposia on calcitonin[68, 68a] provide excellent summaries of the current data. We shall mention briefly only the possible skeletal effects.

Calcitonin produces hypocalcemia and hypophosphatemia by its primary effect, the inhibition of bone resorption. This occurs both in the prevention of the prompt release of calcium from bone by existing cells and in the inhibition of modulation of mesenchymal cells into osteoclasts. The specific site of action in the resorption process is unknown. Calcitonin negates the action of parathyroid hormone on bone. However, it is not specifically an "antiparathyroid hormone" since it also inhibits bone resorption in the absence of parathyroid hormone and does not block parathyroid effects on kidney and gut. The severity of the skeletal manifestations of hyperparathyroidism might be influenced by the calcitonin response of the patient, but in rats, the effect of calcitonin on bone resorption is short lived, and even in the presence of continuous administration of calcitonin, the effect of parathyroid hormone will begin to appear.

In the presence of a low level of turnover in the skeleton due to parathyroidectomy or thyroidectomy, the major skeletal effect of calcitonin is blunted. Conversely, in high resorption states, such as Paget's disease or tumor metastatic to the skeleton, its effect is enhanced. In many animals the hypocalcemic effect of calcitonin decreases with age, and calcitonin is almost without effect on serum calcium levels in normal adult man. This lack of detectable response in serum calcium levels in man is easily explained by the fact that on the average no more than 15 mg of calcium returns from the skeleton to the miscible pool per hour, and even complete suppression of this return would thus reduce the extracellular-fluid calcium only 1.5 per cent one hour after injection. Younger animals, having vastly higher rates of resorption in relation to the total extracellular calcium, naturally exhibit larger effects.

Perhaps the osteopetrosis occurring in the grey-lethal mouse is related to calcitonin excess.[69] In kinetic studies of human osteopetrosis, return of calcium from the skeleton is low. However, in osteopetrosis in man the serum calcium and phosphorus are usually normal. The normal calcium level could be a reflection of increased parathyroid activity in compensation. However, if the normal calcium value in the cases reported by Johnston et al.[70] were due to increased parathyroid activity, one would have expected greater skeletal turnover in the radioactive calcium (^{47}Ca) kinetic studies and an increase in urinary hydroxyproline excretion, neither of which was found. Hypocalcemia has been reported in one group of patients with osteopetrosis[71] in conjunction with a high level of calcitonin activity in the plasma and a marked increase after a calcium infusion. However, in increased calcitonin secretion due to a medullary thyroid carcinoma, despite the presence of hypocalcemia for at least a two-year period, no bone changes were detectable.[72] Thus, the relation between human osteopetrosis and excessive secretion of calcitonin remains unsettled.

Could senile osteoporosis be caused by a decrease in synthesis or release of calcitonin with age or by a reduced effectiveness of normal levels of circulating calcitonin secondary to an increase in inhibiting agents? A plasma heat-labile inhibitor exists,[73] and both theophylline and isoproterenol inhibit the effect of calcitonin, perhaps by increasing cyclic AMP.[74] Decreased calcitonin effect appears unlikely as the cause of postmenopausal or senile osteoporosis since osteoporosis does not develop prematurely or with increased frequency in thyroidectomized patients who are euthyroid after thyroid replacement, nor do they have hypercalcemia. On the other hand, perhaps other tissues, including the parathyroid glands, supply calcitonin in man and meet the requirements following thyroidectomy.[74a]

Whether or not calcitonin is involved in the etiology of osteoporosis, its ability to inhibit bone resorption suggests a role in the therapy of this condition. It reduces bone loss from metastatic deposits of parathyroid carcinoma and lowers the serum calcium levels in hyperparathyroidism, in metastatic tumor and in a large number of experimental situations. Its use in the treatment of senile and postmenopausal osteoporosis by reducing resorption should be studied. Calcitonin could also have an important role in reducing osteoporosis of disuse in a variety of circumstances.

Calcitonin might be effective in the management of carcinoma metastatic to the skeleton, regardless of the source. Since bone destruction at the site of a metastasis is not mediated through the malignant cells directly, but rather is mediated through a change in the functional activity of mesenchymal cells in that area, direct inhibition of bone resorption by calcitonin might reduce or eliminate the lytic activity surrounding metastatic deposits in bone.

Thyroid Hormone

Although changes in thyroid function have profound effects on skeletal remodeling,[75, 76] bone effects of thyroid hormone appear to be part of a general influence on cellular metabolism rather than specifically involved in the day-by-day regulation of skeletal responses. Certainly, bone effects of thyroxin exhibit no feedback influence on thyroid function as exists in the parathyroid-calcitonin loop. Because plasma thyroid hormone levels normally change little during adult life, thyroid hormone is not usually considered to exert a regulatory influence on bone remodeling. Effects from the hormone are usually seen only in thyroid disease.

Hyperthyroidism leads to increased release of calcium from bone secondary to generally increased remodeling, but with proportionately greater resorption than formation. There is a variable elevation of both calcium and phosphorus in the plasma, the urine calcium and hydroxyproline are increased, and negative calcium balance occurs. These changes, which can be produced in hypoparathyroid patients and, hence, appear to be independent of parathyroid hormone,[77] lead to osteoporosis in some patients but are not a major feature of most hyperthyroidism. No correlation exists between this osteoporosis and the other clinical features of the hyperthyroid state. The increased occurrence of osteoid seams in hyperthyroid animals is believed to reflect increased formation rather than osteomalacia.[76]

Hypothyroidism has two important bone effects: a general decrease in structural remodeling and a reduction in bone blood flow. Accretion rates drop to 25 per cent of normal or lower. Formation and resorption surface values are reduced, as is hydroxyproline excretion, and calcium balance does not differ significantly from equilibrium. Hypothyroid patients respond sluggishly to either infused calcium loads, calcitonin or EDTA, almost certainly because the capacity to react to such changes depends upon the resting level of bone turnover and on the bone blood flow, both of which may be limiting in hypothyroidism. Hypothyroid effects are further complicated by such factors as altered gonadal hormone responses and decreased growth hormone release.

Growth Hormone

Aside from its effect on cartilage, growth hormone is a potent stimulus to bone formation. By means of the long-duration, color-coded tetracycline method in adult mature dogs of both sexes, we have shown that growth hormone will produce a substantial increase both in cortical formation and in skeletal mass.[78] The increase is predominantly endosteal, but periosteal and cortical bone formation also rises. A marked increase in trabecular new bone occurs. Although intracortical resorption increases, formation clearly exceeds the increase in resorption and net mass rises. The bone formed is normal in all appearances, histologically and by microradiography. No exostoses occur, and the animals do not become diabetic.

Throughout life, growth hormone is present in the plasma without decrease in normal adults except in one group, postmenopausal females.[79, 80] The combination of intermittent release of human growth hormone (HGH) from the pituitary gland and the short (20 minutes) half-life of growth hormone in the plasma creates a fluctuating pattern of growth hormone level in the plasma. Among the many stimuli to increased release of growth hormone from the pituitary gland are physical activity, estrogens and hypoglycemia. Not only are fasting and hypoglycemia-induced growth hormone levels decreased in postmenopausal women, but these levels can be restored to normal and above normal by estrogens. Estrogens have the same effect of elevating growth hormone in normal adult males.

Comparatively few studies of the effect of growth hormone on adult skeletal-turnover processes have been reported. Accretion has been found to be increased by administration of HGH in normal subjects and in patients with panhypopituitarism.[57] Lafferty[81] described one postmenopausal patient who showed a decrease in accretion and a negative calcium balance when given growth hormone, but treatment was only for two weeks and the kinetic study was done on the third day of hormone administration. As pointed out in Chapter 2, in the section, "Calcium-Kinetic Methods," because of the time lag between matrix formation and mineralization, growth hormone would not be likely to produce an increase in accretion in just three days. In most cases, the increased efficiency of intestinal absorption exceeds the elevation of urinary calcium, and calcium balance is positive.

In contrast with the direct action of HGH on carbohydrate, fat and protein metabolism, its action on epiphyseal cartilage is indirect, requiring the formation of "sulfation factor." Whether the action on new bone formation is direct or indirect is unknown. Given to hypophysectomized rats, growth hormone elevates osteoblastic differentiation and slightly later increases osteoprogenitor cell mitosis.[82] Among its many actions that could influence osteoblastic modulation and osteoblastic function, growth hormone can increase amino acid transport, intracellular protein synthesis, protein synthesis in cell-free preparations, and in the formation of both mRNA and ribosomal RNA.

Gonadal Hormones

Although their effects on skeletal development are known to be different, androgens, estrogens and the synthetic steroids termed *anabolic agents* all appear to act on the adult skeleton in qualitatively the same way. In acute studies these hormones depress bone resorption, with little or no effect on formation. This effect is seen as decreased calcium release from the bone in kinetic studies, with lowered urinary calcium and hydroxyproline, and as positive calcium balance or (as in immobilized or paralyzed patients) reduced negative balance[83] and as a decrease in the elevated bone resorption

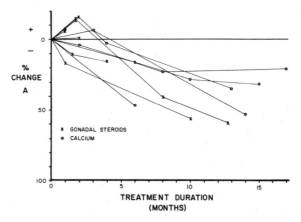

FIGURE 5. Percentage change in accretion (A) from pretreatment levels, plotted as a function of treatment duration, in osteoporotic patients. Data include both our own experience and values recalculated from published material.[85, 86]

surface value.[83a] Calcium absorption from the diet is improved and contributes to the positive balance, but both this change and the decrease in urinary calcium are probably secondary to the primary effect on resorption. In the immature rat resorption of the primary spongiosa is inhibited.[84]

After 6 to 12 months of treatment, in osteoporotic patients accretion is found to be decreased rather than increased,[85, 86] and skeletal balance returns to equilibrium (Fig. 5). Resorption remains at the suppressed level found in the acute studies.

Henneman and Wallach,[87] and Davis et al.[88] have reported on two series of postmenopausal women treated prophylactically with estrogens, and have described decreased rates of loss of height and diminished rates of loss of bone mass in the metacarpal. One study was entirely retrospective, and the other does not include data about its control groups adequate to permit sweeping conclusions. A third such study is reported by Meema and Meema.[88a] These effects are consistent with the observations by Garn et al.[42] and Meema et al.[43] of increased rate of loss of metacarpal and radial cortical bone after the menopause, and suggest that in the premenopausal female estrogen suppresses resorption. After the menopause this suppression is removed, leading to increased resorption, with consequent accelerated bone loss. The influence of estrogen in increasing release of growth hormone may also affect skeletal balance.

Adrenocortical Steroids

Nowhere in the study of skeletal responses is the influence of species specificity more apparent than in the responses to perturbations in circulating levels of adrenocortical steroids. The rabbit becomes markedly osteoporotic when given cortisone,[89] but the intact dog does not, even if very high doses of steroids are used. Increased or decreased density of metaphyseal bone can be produced in rats given exogenous cortical steroids, depending on the calcium and phosphorus intake.[90] The conclusion of Follis[91] that the zone of increased density in the metaphyseal area of cortisone-treated rats as compared with pair-fed controls was due to a decrease in bone resorption was not supported by Sissons and Hadfield.[92]

Nevertheless, the bulk of the data from laboratory animals and from man indicate that the steroids produce an increase in bone resorption, an increase in return of calcium from the skeleton and probably a decrease in formation. In the rabbit there is a prompt rise in bone resorption and a fall in bone formation.[89] There is also bone resorption surrounding vessels in the absence of detectable osteoclasts.

Studies in man are complicated by the fact that only a few patients with spontaneous Cushing's syndrome have been evaluated, normal volunteers have been studied for only comparatively brief periods, and in patients with long-term corticoid therapy, it has been impossible to separate the effects of the treatment from skeletal changes associated with the disease being treated.

The morphometric technics have shown decreased formation surface and increased resorption surface in response to exogenous excess steroid administration.[58] Data from Frost's laboratory indicate a high percentage of resting osteoid seams, little or no tetracycline uptake in most areas, a reduction in formation surface and an increase in resorption surface.[93] Their interpretation was that these data indicated a net *decrease* in both resorption and formation. They reasoned that the net decrease in formation was so severe that the resorption surfaces persisted longer than they would normally. It was postulated that resorption must be diminished, rather than increased, despite the observation of an increase in the amount of resorption surface; otherwise little or no bone at all would remain.

Studies of whole-body kinetics in Cushing's syndrome indicate normal to decreased pool sizes, normal to decreased total pool turnover and usually decreased accretion (approximately 50 per cent of normal).[94, 95] Skeletal release of calcium has not been adequately studied to date, but with subnormal turnover, it would be impossible for calcium release to be more than moderately elevated (see equation 2, Chapter 2).

Short-term use of corticosteroids in usual antiinflammatory doses has not been associated with appreciable change in most kinetic values.[96, 97] Eisenberg and Gordan[94] have reported little change in pool, but slight increases in turnover, urinary calcium and bone accretion. In a series of normal volunteers[97] dexamethasone, 2 mg per day for eight weeks, produced no consistent change in pool, turnover, accretion, skeletal release of calcium or absorption, but did elevate the urine calcium slightly.

Osteoporosis is a usual feature of the spontaneous form of Cushing's syndrome, and urinary calcium tends to be elevated in most such patients, but the degree of elevation is rarely very large and changes in endogenous fecal calcium are small; hence, the discrepancy between bone formation and resorption, although real, does not appear to be as large as the morphometric studies have suggested.

6

METABOLIC BONE DISEASE

Osteomalacia

OSTEOMALACIA, literally "softness of bone," is the skeletal manifestation of one of several metabolic abnormalities that disturb the closely coupled processes of bone-matrix deposition and its mineralization, resulting in both an *increase* in total osteoid tissue present and a *decrease* in the appositional growth rate.[13, 31] The excess osteoid is present as increased numbers of osteoid seams, elevated percentage of total bone surface covered by osteoid, usually but not always increased width of osteoid seams and, probably most important, a rise in the percentage of total skeletal tissue present as osteoid.[101]

The increased osteoid must represent an excess of osteoid formation over matrix mineralization. However, since the appositional growth rate is strikingly reduced, this relative excess of osteoid formation must be associated with a *decreased* rate of osteoid synthesis at each forming surface. At each site the reduction in mineralization exceeds the reduction in matrix formation. This is accompanied by a marked rise in "resting" or inactive osteoid seams, which are not actively mineralizing at all.

Osteomalacias fall into three large categories: those

due to vitamin D deficiency, today most commonly seen in patients with one of the malabsorption syndromes; those associated with hypophosphatemia with normal vitamin D intake, principally familial hypophosphatemia (vitamin-D-resistant rickets), the Fanconi syndrome and renal tubular acidosis; and those associated with defective nucleation without abnormalities of calcium, phosphorus or vitamin D, such as hypophosphatasia and fluoride and strontium intoxication. These groups cannot be distinguished from one another by histologic technics.

Increased numbers of osteoid seams are present in other conditions as well. Paget's disease and hyperthyroidism are high-turnover diseases not characterized by a marked decrease in appositional growth rate or an increase in resting osteoid seams, and therefore do not fall into the osteomalacia group. The increased seam width and decreased appositional growth rate in hypoparathyroidism are associated with a reduction in total osteoid present. Increased osteoid seams are also seen in some cases of hyperparathyroidism with high turnover. Whether these examples reflect just the change in turnover or the effect of disturbances in calcium or phosphorus is not known.

Instead of the normal delay of 5 to 10 days between osteoid synthesis and mineralization, this time lag may become two or three months or longer in some cases of osteomalacia. In addition, important abnormalities can be found in areas that do finally mineralize. These include the persistence of large areas of decreased mineral density and the finding of low mineral content around many osteocytes.[102-104] Tetracycline given *in vivo* and many stains used *in vitro* show abnormal localization patterns suggesting both persisting abnormalities of mineralization and increased reactivity of these regions of bone.

There is probably no bone disorder in which the results of kinetic studies have been so diverse and so hard to evaluate. In most cases both the exchangeable pool and the rates of accretion and calcium return have been elevated, sometimes greatly. But in a few cases, both vitamin-D-deficient and vitamin-D-resistant kinetic values have been normal or low.[105, 106] There seem to be no clinical or biochemical features distinguishing these patterns, and unfortunately almost no cases have been studied simultaneously by morphometric and kinetic methods. One uniform finding, however, in all types studied, and regardless of the original kinetic values, has been the response to effective treatment, namely, an increase in mineral accretion rate. Similarly, widely divergent values have been reported from morphometric studies. In the ribs of 14 patients with osteomalacia of diverse etiology, Arnstein et al.[13] report five cases with increased, five with decreased and four with normal bone formation.

There has been serious question about whether a finding of high mineral accretion can be taken seriously in osteomalacia, a disease characterized by a disorder in nucleation and mineralization.[107] Poorly mineralized bone, particularly around osteocytes, may exchange more readily than usual with the plasma, thus explaining both the large pool and the elevated accretion rate. On the other hand, the rate of bone formation will depend upon the product of the increased number of forming surfaces and the decreased average rate of mineralization at each surface. We suggest that the occasional reports of low accretion values reflect periods of relative or absolute nucleation arrest, and the more usually found high values represent the product of slow mineralization at a large number of sites or excessive long-term exchange in poorly mineralized regions of bone (or both).

The common notion is that osteomalacia is characterized by calcium deficiency and mineral-hungry bone, and is associated with defective calcium absorption from the intestinal lumen and high retention of infused calcium loads. To a certain extent, all three notions are true, but unfortunately they tend to obscure rather than to illuminate the issue. Rachitic cartilage *is* mineral-hungry and will readily mineralize *in vitro* in normal plasma, but osteomalacic osteoid fails to do so. The reason is that it has not yet been nucleated. On histochemical examination the characteristic premineralization changes in osteoid are uniformly absent,[8] with a return of these features on effective treatment, even before the plasma mineral levels change. Furthermore, poor intestinal absorption in laboratory animals produces osteoporosis, not osteomalacia, and only under extreme conditions of deprivation in growing young animals does a rachitic lesion develop. Indeed, as is well known, the standard rachitogenic diet in the rat is deficient in phosphorus, not calcium. Finally, using high retention of infused calcium loads to diagnose osteomalacia and to distinguish it from osteoporosis, as some investigators[108] have done, is an example of circular reasoning. If osteomalacic osteoid will not mineralize *in vitro,* it is not likely to do so when the calcium is added *in vivo,* particularly when the characteristic plasma calcium of osteomalacia is already normal or only minimally depressed. The high retention probably represents suppression of bone resorption by the transient induced hypercalcemia.

What then, if not calcium deficiency, is the reason for delayed mineralization? Extracellular enzymatic processes under osteoblast control must be necessary to prepare the matrix to receive mineral. An inherited enzymatic deficiency, such as hypophosphatasia, might act by leading to defective matrix maturation. Similarly, bone intoxication by substances such as fluoride can be thought of as interfering with maturation.

Both hypophosphatasia and fluoride intoxication are rare and may have their principal importance as models of the commoner causes of osteomalacia. Phosphate deficiency alone or together with vitamin D deficiency may adversely affect osteoblast competence in some similar way. By far the majority of cases of osteomalacia are characterized by severe hypophosphatemia, and it is now recognized that phosphate deficiency can cause profound cellular dysfunction.[109]

The osteoblast is likely to be more phosphate-deficient than the average somatic cell. In normal extracellular fluid there is an excess of phosphate in relation to calcium (with respect to their molar ratios in hydroxyapatite), but when plasma phosphate drops below 2 mg per 100 ml, phosphate becomes limiting, and the nucleated matrix may be expected to sweep the environment of almost all the available phosphate. Thus, the environment of an osteoblast may be expected to be more phosphate-depleted than that of other tissues.

It cannot be stated with certainty that hypophosphatemia is responsible for osteoblast dysfunction, but such an explanation has many attractive features, not least of which are the response to phosphate treatment[106] and the fact of identical histochemical abnormalities in the matrix of both vitamin-D-deficient and vitamin-D-resistant osteomalacia.[8]

Osteoporosis

Definition

Osteoporosis is the condition of the skeleton or a part of the skeleton in which the bone present per unit volume is decreased in amount but normal in composition. This decrease is relative to a "normal" value: to ascertain the effects of age-related changes, "normal" controls must be drawn from the group 25 to 35 years old with maximum skeletal mass. To determine the effects of factors other than age, the "normal" controls must be age-matched.

Although there may be subtle morphologic changes in bone composition in the osteoporoses, there is little doubt that a sufficient reduction in bone mass can adequately account for the fragility of osteoporotic bone, which is, after all, its only important consequence. We now recognize that the osteoporoses are a heterogeneous group of disorders that may develop at any rate of bone remodeling from high to low. Since coupling usually exists between formation and resorption, the emphasis in any osteoporosis has to be on forces that maintain resorption at a higher level than formation regardless of the absolute rate of either. This characterization of osteoporosis is unabashedly nonspecific, and includes osteoporoses of diverse etiology most of which have nothing in common except their end result.

Corticosteroid Osteoporosis

Osteoporosis regularly occurs in Cushing's syndrome, and on biopsy is associated with striking reductions in bone-forming surface and appositional growth rate. Resorption surface is markedly increased.[58] Although conflicting data exist concerning an increase or decrease in resorption (as discussed in Chapter 5 in the section "Adrenocortical Steroids"), clinical observations suggest that resorption is actually elevated. In the full-blown syndrome, formation seems to be reduced so completely that there is nowhere to store calcium during dietary absorption, and hence even the minimal loss characteristic of the postabsorptive phase cannot be offset. Any resorptive stimulation above that minimal level would simply accelerate the process still more.

Local Osteoporoses

A special group of local osteoporoses is associated with immobilization and disuse, denervation, fracture, inflammation and trauma. The sequence of remodeling changes evoked by denervation or tendon section[57, 57a] is first a large increase in resorption together with a transient slight reduction in formation, followed by a phase of enhanced formation and still greater resorption. This is ultimately succeeded by gradual reduction first in resorption and then in formation. Again, resorption and formation are seen to be closely coupled. After the initial reduction in stress, resorption leads and formation follows, with a lag period varying from a few days in small animals to a few weeks in dogs and man. Resorption is enhanced first and subsides first, whereas formation is elevated after the lag phase and subsides last. In other words, this is a "high-turnover osteoporosis." A corollary to these sequential changes is the fact that, depending on how soon one studies the process, one can find virtually any combination of formation-resorption effects representing various stages in the evolution of the process, but not necessarily reflecting the direct effects of mechanical forces.

Similarly, bones near a fracture, even if separated by a joint, show a high uptake of ^{47}Ca for months after the injury, and this is true even while they are demonstrably osteoporotic.[110] Some have argued that the neural and vascular changes produced indirectly in these experiments are more responsible for the remodeling changes than the immobilization per se, but exactly the same sequence of changes is seen with simple casting of a limb,[56] and it seems probable that the withdrawal of tonic muscle pulls and of weight-bearing stresses, by whatever mechanism, evokes essentially similar responses.

Bone around inflamed joints also becomes osteoporotic. Kinetic measurements based on local uptake data indicate an average accretion value at least twice as high as normal.[97] This, too, seems to be a high-turnover osteoporosis.

Space Flight Osteoporosis

With its unique combination of weightlessness, increased corticosteroid release, restraint, reduced exercise and altered dietary intake, space flight presents a particularly complex problem in loss of skeletal mass. Wide variations in the amount of loss exist among the astronauts, and even greater differences have been reported from separate skeletal sites from the same astronaut.[110a, 110b] Further detailed study of skeletal renewal under conditions existing in orbital flight will be vital to the space program.

Senile and Postmenopausal Osteoporoses

Senile and postmenopausal osteoporoses probably affect at least 4,000,000 to 6,000,000 women in the

United States. The true prevalence is undoubtedly even higher because clinical roentgenograms are admittedly a crude measure of disease.[111, 112] A decrease of 30 to 50 per cent in skeletal mass is required for clinical detection of osteoporosis in the lumbar spine. Fractures of the hip, radius, humerus, vertebrae, and ribs secondary to osteoporosis constitute a major health hazard among the elderly.

Difficulties in the study of these conditions are based on three factors. The first is the low order of magnitude of the changes involved. Loss of only 30 mg of calcium per day for 30 years results in a 30 per cent loss in skeletal mass. The second difficulty is the fact that the progress of osteoporosis is nonlinear with respect to time.[113] The third complexity deals with the inability to measure skeletal mass accurately. In many kinetic studies the values for accretion and for return of calcium from the skeleton have been compared with similar values obtained from young normal persons, whose skeletal mass may be 30 per cent greater. The presence of a "normal" accretion value for a skeleton that has a 30 per cent decrease in mass would actually indicate an increase in accretion per gram of bone.

Three major questions remain unanswered. The first is why a universal age-related loss of skeletal mass occurs. The second is why the rate of loss of skeletal mass is accelerated in postmenopausal females. And the third is whether the patients who show *clinical* manifestation of this universal process are different by virtue of other abnormalities superimposed upon the usual age-related bone loss or represent those who started with a lower initial bone mass and have lost bone for a longer time.

Patients with clinically manifest postmenopausal

osteoporosis have been clearly shown to have much less bone than age-matched controls.[114] They exhibit a different steroid-excretion response to ACTH,[80] a depressed growth-hormone response to insulin-induced hypoglycemia and possibly also a depressed intestinal calcium-absorption efficiency.[115]

The focus of investigation must be on the imbalance between formation and resorption that leads to loss of bone. The first clear formulation of this imbalance between formation and resorption was the well-known hypothesis of Fuller Albright and his collaborators,[116] to the effect that all osteoporoses were caused by a primary decrease in osteoblast activity, without a corresponding reduction in bone resorption. Like all useful hypotheses, it served its purpose well by integrating existing knowledge and by making predictions that could be experimentally tested. The first such test was provided by calcium tracer studies, such as those summarized in Figure 6. The majority of such studies have shown that, taken as a group, patients with postmenopausal or senile osteoporosis have essentially the same rate of calcium turnover as normal persons.[117-119] Urinary calcium and endogenous fecal calcium have also been shown to be normal in these patients; hence, total skeletal accretion is within normal limits as well. However, in all kinetic studies in postmenopausal osteoporosis, resorption has also been found to be within the normal range. In most such studies return of calcium from the skeleton has exceeded accretion in the order of 50 to 100 mg per day. Hence, whereas accretion and calcium return from the skeleton and turnover are all technically "normal," the difference between them is not, and a net loss of this magnitude is compatible with the rate of progression of the disorder. Once again this

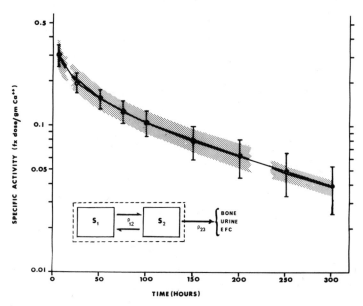

FIGURE 6. Average values for plasma calcium specific activity in 14 untreated osteoporotic patients, superimposed on a composite reference curve.[27] Both sets of data have been normalized to 1.7 m² of body-surface area. The solutions of the two-compartment analysis of the mean values for each group are contained in the inset. The symbols in the inset have the following meaning: S_1 and S_2 represent the mass of the slow and fast compartments, respectively, of the miscible calcium pool; ρ_{12} represents the flux between these two compartments (the intercompartmental flux), and ρ_{23} the movement of calcium out of both compartments to bone, urine and feces (external turnover) as described in Chapter 2 in the section "Calcium-Kinetic Methods." Data from calcium-kinetic studies in osteoporotic patients do not deviate from the range of age-related normal values.

problem involves the question of what is normal. Thus far, kinetic studies in adults have failed to demonstrate any consistent change in accretion or removal with age, and these patients with osteoporosis are said to have "normal" values with reference to standard adult levels, corrected for differences in body size. But bone mass is decreased in osteoporosis, and hence accretion and removal rates, expressed per unit bone mass, must be considered to be elevated rather than normal. On the other hand, in the context of calcium homeostasis, it is the size of the body, not the size of the skeleton, that is important. Hence, skeletal turnover is elevated if expressed per unit bone mass, but normal if expressed per unit body mass. Also, the larger number of lowly mineralized osteons in the aged[4] or the increase in total bone surface may change the proportion of the accretion value that is due to long-term exchange.

Soon after the publication of the first mineral tracer studies, Jowsey[4] and Frost,[33] employing morphometric methods, showed the percentage of bone-forming surface to be normal or high and resorption surface to be markedly elevated, and suggested that osteoporosis was a disease of resorption. Since the total surface existing in osteoporotic bone is much increased over that in normal bone, even a normal "percentage surface" figure for a patient with osteoporosis would represent substantially more surface having a resorption or formation appearance. Quantitative studies from Frost's laboratory of appositional growth rate and numbers of new osteons formed per year in rib-biopsy samples from osteoporotic patients[120] indicate that, although the number of bone-forming sites is extremely variable, the values are predominantly low and the average rate of bone formation at each of them is reduced. At least some of this reduction is due to long periods of functional arrest, during which the osteoblasts do nothing at all, and it is not known whether, while active, they work more or less efficiently than normal. (The similarity of this observation to the central feature of the Albright hypothesis will not be missed.) Morphometric studies[36] suggest subnormal Haversian resorption but excessive endosteal resorption rates, and so it would seem that all the cellular processes involved in renewal are disturbed in these samples. These data on ribs cannot safely be extended to the entire skeleton, but these observations concerning changes in cell function may be important.

Despite these uncertainties with the kinetic and morphometric technics, extremely important advances in the understanding of osteoporosis have occurred in the last decade. The first of these was the demonstration that the age-related loss of bone mass is not confined to the axial skeleton, and is a universal process, involving all races and both sexes.[42] The fact that the age-related loss begins before the menopause in the female and is present in the male indicates that it is not simply a postmenopausal phenomenon. On the other hand, substantial data indicate clearly that postmenopausal osteoporosis is a separate category from senile osteoporosis and that the menopause exerts an important additive influence superimposed on the universal age-related loss.

In summary, the various methods for measuring skeletal renewal reveal, in postmenopausal and senile osteoporosis, that calcium turnover, total skeletal accretion and return of calcium from the skeleton are "normal" in relation to body weight but increased in relation to skeletal mass; that bone forming surface is elevated; that bone resorption surface is markedly elevated; and that, at least in some regions, the rate of cellular activity on these surfaces is reduced. What do these observations tell us about the pathogenesis of the disorder?

A number of possible mechanisms of development of senile and postmenopausal osteoporosis warrant consideration. Some involve primary decrease in formation, and others, increased resorption, but in each the central question must be how resorption is *consistently* maintained at levels higher than formation.

The decrease in appositional growth rate with age raises the possibility of a decrease in osteoblastic function or a reduction in modulation from osteoprogenitor cells to osteoblasts. The rate of skeletal loss is accelerated in postmenopausal women, the one group showing a decrease in resting levels of growth hormone and a decrease in growth-hormone response to hypoglycemia.[79, 80] Our finding that this hormone both reverses the endosteal loss of cortical bone in the intact adult animal and stimulates bone formation[78] reinforces the suggestion that it may be another factor in the complex process controlling net skeletal balance.

Although calcium deficiency can produce osteoporosis in a number of laboratory animals, proof that dietary deficiency causes human osteoporosis is lacking. Average dietary intakes in osteoporotic patients are lower than normal,[121] but not by much, and whereas low intakes may be a major factor in a few patients, they cannot be implicated in the majority. Furthermore, available epidemiologic studies indicate no difference between the age-related loss of bone in populations with high and low dietary calcium intake.[42] However, at least some of these studies have specifically excluded known osteoporotic patients; these patients may be osteoporotic precisely because they are not "normal" with respect to factors such as dietary calcium requirements.

Nevertheless, it seems more reasonable to propose that the significance of calcium-deficiency osteoporosis lies not in direct translation into a clinical situation, but in the reminder that calcium homeostasis, mediated by parathyroid hormone, is perfectly capable of maintaining resorption in excess of formation. Hormone levels need not be excessive to produce this result, provided that bone responsiveness to the hormone is enhanced relative to the response of other PTH end organs. Certainly, increased responsiveness locally appears to underlie the development of disuse osteoporosis. Heaney[122] has proposed that a similar mechanism is operative in postmenopausal osteoporosis, and under these circumstances, net skeletal loss would occur at normal or lower than normal levels of endogenous parathyroid activity.

It may seem paradoxical to propose that decreased PTH secretion could lead to an excess of resorption over formation, and it would be, if it were not for the other end-organ effects of PTH, namely, intestinal absorption and renal tubular reabsorption. If we exclude intestinal effects by considering only the fasting organism, resorption is seen to exceed formation by an amount equal to the urinary calcium excretion. Since, at normal filtered loads, PTH is a major determinant of excretion, it follows that the urinary calcium, and hence the postabsorptive excess of resorption over formation, will be *inversely* related to the circulating PTH level. Thus, if the response of bone to PTH is enhanced in relation to the other PTH end organs, calcium homeostasis will be maintained at a lower level of PTH, and the postabsorptive excess of bone resorption will be increased rather than decreased.

Consistent with the notion of decreased endogenous PTH is the fact that plasma phosphate is higher in postmenopausal women, particularly in castrates,[123] and that the level of plasma phosphate can be directly correlated with the severity of the osteoporosis.[124] It is recognized that many factors other than PTH affect the plasma phosphate, but until a suitable assay for low and normal levels of human PTH is developed, such indirect evidence of decreased endogenous PTH is all that is available.

Additional evidence has accumulated to support the notion that bone resorptive response to PTH is strongly dependent on a whole host of environmental factors. We have already indicated that agents such as oxygen and heparin enhance resorptive response, whereas estrogens, fluoride, exercise, phosphate and even calcium itself depress resorption in the presence of a fixed level of PTH. Estrogen withdrawal at the menopause and the general decrease in physical activity with aging provide two nearly universal factors consistent both with a heightened responsiveness to endogenous PTH and with the known decrease in bone mass in aging women.

Experience with Treatment

Gonadal hormone therapy has been the mainstay of treatment for the past 25 years, and calcium supplements have been added during the past 10. Despite the fact that these agents decrease resorption, and hence ought to favor positive bone balance, almost without exception they have failed to increase bone mass in osteoporotic patients. They routinely produce positive calcium balance in acute studies, but months or years later they have produced no x-ray evidence of increased bone density. This failure has usually been explained by the claim that x-ray examination was too insensitive to detect the real changes, or by allusion to a large systematic error in the balance technic to the effect that the patients were not really in positive balance in the first place. Neither explanation is satisfying. Only a few careful follow-up studies of long-term treatment have been published, and these have shown that, after 8 to 12 months of continuous treatment, patients are no longer in positive calcium balance. Furthermore, kinetic studies in the same patients, such as those in Figure 5, reveal a roughly 40 per cent reduction in mineral accretion beginning sometime after the sixth month of therapy. In other words, treatment has reduced resorption, and the organism has responded by reducing formation to match! Positive balance is confined to the interval when the one is catching up with the other. This is one more striking example of coupling between these two processes in bone.

Neither the homeostatic nor the piezoelectrical coupling mechanisms discussed earlier adequately explain this example of the phenomenon, for in the homeostatic scheme, formation is not a controlled variable, and the bone mass change is obviously inadequate to reduce the formation stimulus of the mechanical-piezoelectrical scheme. Another coupling mechanism must be sought.

Nevertheless, the data on the increased rate of skeletal loss after the menopause and the decrease in loss after estrogen administration (discussed in Chapter 5, under the heading "Gonadal Hormones") support the notion that all postmenopausal osteoporotic women should receive estrogen substitution therapy. If additional controlled studies substantiate the work of Davis et al.[88] and Meema and Meema,[88a] probably all postmenopausal women should be treated unless some contraindication exists.

Phosphate, fluoride and calcitonin are additional

potentially useful agents, and all three act in part by depressing resorption. To date, their long-term effects in the treatment of human osteoporosis are unknown. At high doses fluoride can increase skeletal mass, but it does so by inducing abnormal bone production. The role of long-duration, low-dose schedules is currently under investigation. Fluoride-loaded animals are protected against heparin-induced osteoporosis,[125] and require an excessive osteoclast response to mobilize a standard amount of calcium.[52]

It is also interesting that the only investigator reporting consistently positive calcium balance and increased bone density with calcium treatment has been Nordin,[126] who employed, not the calcium preparations commonly used in the United States, but calcium *glycerophosphate*. To the extent that these effects were real, one must speculate whether they were not due more to the phosphate than to the calcium. Finally, the importance of activity in reducing resorption must be stressed.

Growth hormone is interesting not because it diminishes the rate of loss but, as we have shown, because it directly stimulates new bone formation when given to adult dogs under controlled conditions. To our knowledge no other agent, with the exception of fluoride given in high dosage, has the same effect.

Parathyroid Disorders

The physiologic significance of the parathyroid glands lies in calcium homeostasis, and the principal effect of parathyroid disorders is clearly on the regulation of calcium ion concentration. Bone changes are of only secondary clinical importance, but they are noteworthy in the context of this monograph because of what they reveal about parathyroid effects on skeletal renewal.

In surgical or idiopathic hypoparathyroidism bone remodeling is reduced by at least 75 per cent. Bone formation and resorption surfaces are markedly reduced, but the linear apposition rate on the reduced number of forming surfaces remains normal.[27] Accretion rates are only about 25 per cent of normal.[20] Since this value still contains some element of long-term exchange with the diffuse component of bone, true bone formation is probably reduced even more than is apparent from such figures. Plainly, parathyroid hormone is the principal determinant of the quantity of skeletal turnover in the adult. This effect is probably exerted primarily on the resorptive process, changes in formation being secondary (that is, one more manifestation of the coupling between resorption and formation).

As is not surprising, hyperparathyroid states are associated with evidence of increased skeletal remodeling. Jowsey[127] noted that resorption surfaces were markedly increased in all her cases of hyperparathyroidism, even those with only mild hypercalcemia and without clinical or roentgenographic evidence of bone disease. Formation surfaces were increased in only 4 of 26 cases.[34] Total body kinetic measurements have usually shown increased pools, turnover, accretion and return, with the extent of the change correlating fairly well with the degree of elevation of the plasma calcium and with the presence of demonstrable bone involvement.[94, 119] In contrast with the morphologic studies, some patients are found to have kinetic values within normal limits— an interesting and possibly illuminating dissociation.

Many patients with mild hyperparathyroidism fail to

have very negative calcium balances, and lose total bone mass fairly slowly. In such patients the dissociated formation and resorption surface figures seen on biopsy cannot be translated directly into corresponding disparate rates of formation and resorption.

A similar disparity has already been noted in the data derived from biopsies in patients with postmenopausal osteoporosis. There are only a few ways in which this apparent disagreement between the balance kinetic data and the surface data can be resolved. In the first place, the actual magnitude of the skeletal turnover may be so much lower than the present kinetic methods suggest (for example, 50 to 100 mg per day) that even a twofold difference between resorption and formation surface would be compatible with the observed small degree of negative calcium balance. Secondly, the linear resorption rate may be reduced in relation to the normal so that an increase in surface need not mean a corresponding increase in rate of resorption. And, finally, the "turn-around time" may be prolonged[128] so that much of the resorption surface would be completely inactive at the time of the biopsy, resorption having been completed and new formation having not yet begun.

The explanation for the difference between hyperparathyroid patients with and without bone disease may be found in the presence of normal compensatory mechanisms capable of offsetting moderate parathyroid hormone excesses. Thus, calcitonin secretion may be able to keep pace with the autonomous parathyroid gland and counteract its resorptive effect in bone. Calcitonin has a prompt hypocalcemic effect generally considered to reflect suppression of resorption by existing osteoclasts and osteocytes, and in longer studies it decreases the modulation of resting cells into osteoclasts. Decreased modulation of this type, however, is not a sufficient explanation for the effects of hyperparathyroidism, for osteoclasts are increased, as is the resorption surface. Consequently, only by direct inhibitory effect of osteoclastic function (that is, linear resorption rate) would a calcitonin effect be useful in accounting for the discrepancy between the two methods. Baylink and co-workers[129] have recently shown that calcitonin has precisely this effect on endosteal resorption in the rat.

In addition, hypercalcemia itself has been demonstrated to reduce hydroxyproline release from bone in response to fixed levels of parathyroid hormone,[48] and hence there are at least two mechanisms capable of explaining the dissociation between resorption rates and resorption surface in hyperparathyroidism.

Pseudohypoparathyroidism has fascinated investigators for years because of the apparent resistance to parathyroid hormone found in this disorder. There is no question of deficiency of parathyroid hormone in this condition. The hormone has been identified in plasma from pseudohypoparathyroid patients. In addition, the original flurry of interest in a possible role of calcitonin, based on the finding of extremely high calcitonin levels in the thyroid gland of these patients, has subsided with the failure to find calcitonin in the plasma and the failure of patients to respond to thyroidectomy. Jowsey[127] and Takahashi, Frost and Kuhn[128] have recently shown normal or increased resorption surfaces in bone from patients with pseudohypoparathyroidism. However, linear resorption rates could not be determined, and thus it is not possible to say whether actual bone resorption will be in the hypoparathyroid or the euparathyroid range. Nevertheless, this finding represents a clear difference from the parathyroprivic disorders, and suggests an abnormality in osteoclast competence.

REFERENCES

1. Nagant de Deuxchaisnes, C., and Krane, S. M. Paget's disease of bone: clinical and metabolic observations. *Medicine* 43:233–266, 1964.
1a. Ham, A. W. *Histology*. Sixth edition. Philadelphia: Lippincott, 1969.
2. Johnson, L. C. Morphologic analysis in pathology: kinetics of disease and general biology of bone. In Henry Ford Hospital International Symposium. *Bone Biodynamics*. Edited by H. M. Frost. Boston: Little, Brown, 1964. Pp. 543–654.
3. Cohen, J., and Harris, W. H. Three-dimensional anatomy of Haversian systems. *J. Bone & Joint Surg.* 40A:419–434, 1958.
4. Jowsey, J. Age changes in human bone. *Clin. Orthop.* 17:210–218, 1960.
5. Young, R. W. Control of cell specialization in bone. *Clin. Orthop.* 45:153–156, 1966.
6. Kashiwa, H. K. Glyoxal bis (2-hydroxyanil) method for differential staining of intracellular calcium in bone. In International Congress Series. No. 159. *Parathyroid Hormone and Thyrocalcitonin (Calcitonin): Proceedings of the third Parathyroid Conference: Montreal, Canada, October 16–20, 1967.* Edited by R. V. Talmage and L. F. Bélanger. Co-editor: I. Clark. Amsterdam C, Netherlands: Excerpta Medica, 1968. P. 198.
7. Marshall, J. H., White, V. K., and Cohen, J. Microscopic metabolism of calcium in bone. I. Three-dimensional deposition of Ca^{45} in canine osteons. *Radiation Research* 10:197–212, 1959. Marshall, J. H., Rowland, R. E., and Jowsey, J. II. Quantitative autoradiography. *Ibid.* 10:213–233, 1959. *Idem.* III. Microangiographic measurements of mineral density. *Ibid.* 10:234–242, 1959. *Idem.* IV. Ca^{45} deposition and growth rate in canine osteons. *Ibid.* 10:243–257, 1959. *Idem.* V. Paradox of diffuse activity and long-term exchange. *Ibid.* 10:258–270, 1959.
8. Johnson, L. C. Kinetics of skeletal remodeling. In *Structural Organization of the Skeleton: A symposium.* (Birth Defects Original Article Series.) Edited by D. Bergsma. New York: The National Foundation, 1966. Vol. 2 (1), pp. 66–142.
9. Irving, J. T., and Wuthier, R. E. Histochemistry and biochemistry of calcification with special references to role of lipids. *Clin. Orthop.* 56:237–260, 1968.

References

10. Glimcher, M. J., and Krane, S. M. Organization and structure of bone and mechanism of calcification. In *Treatise on Collagen*. Edited by G. N. Ramachandran and B. S. Gould. Vol. 2. Part B. London: Academic Press, 1968. Pp. 68–251.

10a. Pellegrino, E. D., and Biltz, R. M. Bone carbonate and the Ca to P molar ratio. *Nature* (London) 219:1261–1262, 1968.

10b. Biltz, R. M., and Pellegrino, E. D. The chemical anatomy of bone. I. A comparative study of bone composition in sixteen vertebrates. *J. Bone & Joint Surg.* 51A:456–466, 1969.

11. Neuman, W. F., and Neuman, M. W. *The Chemical Dynamics of Bone Mineral*. Chicago: Univ. of Chicago Press, 1958.

12. Glimcher, M. J. Molecular biology of mineralized tissues with particular reference to bone. *Rev. Mod. Physics* 31:359–393, 1959.

12a. Fleisch, H., Maerki, J., and Russell, R. G. G. Effect of pyrophosphate on dissolution of hydroxyapatite and its possible importance in calcium homeostasis. *Proc. Soc. Exper. Biol. & Med.* 22:317–320, 1966.

12b. Avioli, L. V., McDonald, J. E., Henneman, P. H., and Lee, S. W. Relationship of parathyroid activity to pyrophosphate excretion. *J. Clin. Investigation* 45:1093–1102, 1966.

12c. Posen, S. Alkaline phosphatase. *Ann. Int. Med.* 67:183–203, 1967.

13. Arnstein, A. R., Frame, B., and Frost, H. M. Recent progress in osteomalacia and rickets. *Ann. Int. Med.* 67:1296–1330, 1967.

14. Gaillard, P. J. Parathyroid and bone in tissue culture. In Symposium on Advances in Parathyroid Research. Rice University, 1960. *The Parathyroids: Proceedings*. Edited by R. O. Greep and R. V. Talmage. Springfield, Illinois: Thomas, 1961. Pp. 20–48.

15. Goldhaber, P. Bone resorption factors, cofactors and giant vacuole osteoclasts in tissue culture. In *The Parathyroid Glands: Ultrastructure, secretion, and function: With an introduction by F. C. McLean*. Edited by P. J. Gaillard, R. V. Talmage and A. M. Budy. Chicago, Illinois: Univ. of Chicago Press, 1965. Pp. 153–169.

15a. Neuman, W. F., Mulryan, B. J., and Martin, G. R. Chemical view of osteoclasis based on studies with yttrium. *Clin. Orthop.* 17:124–134, 1960.

16. Gaillard, P. J. Personal communication, 1967.

17. Bélanger, L. F., Robichon, J., Migicovsky, B. B., Copp, D. H., and Vincent, J. Resorption without osteoclasts (osteolysis). In *Mechanisms of Hard Tissue Destruction*. Edited by R. F. Sognnaes. Washington, D. C.: American Association for the Advancement of Science, 1963. P. 531.

18. Bélanger, L. F., and Robichon, J. Parathormone-induced osteolysis in dogs: microradiographic and alpharadiographic survey. *J. Bone & Joint Surg.* 46A:1008–1012, 1964.

19. Bauer, G. C. H., Carlsson, A., and Lindquist, B. Evaluation of accretion, resorption, and exchange reactions in the skeleton. *K. Fysiogr. Sallskapets Lundi Förhandl.* 25:3–18, 1955.

19a. Bauer, G. C. H. Tracer techniques for study of bone metabolism in man. *Advances in Biol. Med. Phys.* 10:227–275, 1965.

20. Heaney, R. P., and Whedon, G. D. Radiocalcium studies of bone formation rate in human metabolic bone disease. *J. Clin. Endocrinol. & Metab.* 18:1246–1267, 1958.

21. Aubert, J. P., and Milhaud, G. Méthode de mesure des principales voies du métabolisme calcique chez l'homme. *Biochem. et Biophys. Acta* 39:122–139, 1960.

22. Marshall, J. H. Radioactive hotspots, bone growth and bone cancer: self-burial of calcium-like hotspots. In Symposium on Radioisotopes and Bone. Princeton, New Jersey, 1960. *Radioisotopes and Bone.* Edited under direction of F. C. McLean by P. Lacroix and A. M. Budy. Oxford: Blackwell Scientific Publications, 1962. Pp. 35–50.

23. Rowland, R. E. Personal communication, 1968.

24. Neer, R., Berman, M., Fisher, L., and Rosenberg, L. E. Multicompartmental analysis of calcium kinetics in normal adult males. *J. Clin. Investigation* 46:1364–1379, 1967.

25. Heaney, R. P. Evaluation and interpretation of calcium-kinetic data in man. *Clin. Orthop.* 31:153–183, 1963.

25a. Solomon, A. K. Compartmental methods of kinetic analysis. Chapter 5. In *Mineral Metabolism: An advanced treatise.* Edited by C. L. Comar and F. Bronner. Vol. 1. Part A. New York: Academic Press, 1960. Pp. 119–167.

26. DeGrazia, J. A., Ivanovich, P., Fellows, H., and Rich, C. Double isotope method for measurement of intestinal absorption of calcium in man. *J. Lab. & Clin. Med.* 66:822–829, 1965.

27. Heaney, R. P., et al. Normal reference standard for radiocalcium turnover and excretion in humans. *J. Lab. & Clin. Med.* 64:21–28, 1964.

28. Pirok, D. J., Ramser, J. R., Takahashi, H., Villanueva, A. R., and Frost, H. M. Normal histological, tetracycline and dynamic parameters in human, mineralized bone sections. *Henry Ford Hospital M. Bull.* 14:195–218, 1966.

29. Harris, W. H. Microscopic method of determining rates of bone growth. *Nature* (London) 188:1038, 1960.

30. Jowsey, J., et al. Quantitative microradiographic studies of normal and osteoporotic bone. *J. Bone & Joint Surg.* 47A:785–806, 1965.

31. Kelly, P. J., Jowsey, J., and Riggs, B. L. Comparison of different morphologic methods of determining bone formation. *Clin. Orthop.* 40:7–11, 1965.

32. Harris, W. H., Jackson, R. H., and Jowsey, J. *In vivo* distribution of tetracyclines in canine bone. *J. Bone & Joint Surg.* 44A:1308–1320, 1962.

33. Frost, H. M. Postmenopausal osteoporosis: disturbance in osteoclasia. *J. Am. Geriatric Soc.* 9:1078–1085, 1961.

34. Riggs, B. L., Kelly, P. J., Jowsey, J., and Keating, R. Skeletal alterations in hyperparathyroidism: determination of bone formation, resorption and morphologic changes by microradiography. *J. Clin. Endocrinol. & Metab.* 25:777–783, 1965.

References

35. Lee, W. R., Marshall, J. H., and Sissons, H. A.   Calcium accretion and bone formation in dogs: experimental comparison between results of Ca-45 kinetic analysis and tetracycline labelling. *J. Bone & Joint Surg.* 47B:157–180, 1965.

35a. Baylink, D., Stauffer, M., Wergedal, J., and Rich, C.   Formation, mineralization and resorption of bone in vitamin D deficiency. In press.

36. Wu, K., Jett, S., and Frost, H. M.   Bone resorption rates in rib in physiological, senile, and postmenopausal osteoporoses. *J. Lab. & Clin. Med.* 69:810–818, 1967.

37. Kelly, P. J.   Bone remodeling in puppies with experimental rickets. *J. Lab. & Clin. Med.* 70:94–105, 1967.

38. Jowsey, J.   Personal communication, 1967.

39. Harris, W. H., Haywood, E. A., Lavorgna, J., and Hamblen, D. L.   Spatial and temporal variations in cortical bone formation in dogs: long-term study. *J. Bone & Joint Surg.* 50A:1118–1128, 1968.

40. Prockop, D. J., and Kivirikko, K. I.   Review: relationship of hydroxyproline excretion in urine to collagen metabolism: biochemistry and clinical applications. *Ann. Int. Med.* 66:1243–1266, 1967.

41. Pechet, M. M., Bobadilla, E., Carroll, E. L., and Hesse, R. H.   Regulation of bone resorption and formation: influences of thyrocalcitonin, parathyroid hormone, neutral phosphate, and vitamin D_3. *Am. J. Med.* 43:696–710, 1967.

42. Garn, S. M., Rohmann, C. G., and Wagner, B.   Bone loss as general phenomenon in man. *Federation Proc.* 26:1729–1736, 1967.

43. Meema, H. E., Bunker, M. L., and Meema, S.   Loss of compact bone due to menopause. *Obst. & Gynec.* 26:333–343, 1965.

44. Sorenson, J. A., and Cameron, J. R.   Reliable *in vivo* measurement of bone-mineral content. *J. Bone & Joint Surg.* 49A:481–497, 1967.

45. Isaksson, B., and Sjögren, B.   Critical evaluation of mineral and nitrogen balances in man. *Proc. Nutrition Soc.* 26:106–116, 1967.

46. Rundo, J.   Retention of Barium-133 in man. *Internat. J. Radiat. Biol.* 13:301, 1967.

46a. Harrison, G. E., Carr, T. E. F., and Sutton, A.   Distribution of radioactive calcium, strontium, barium, and radium following intravenous injection into healthy man. *Internat. J. Radiat. Biol.* 13:235–247, 1967.

47. Rose, G. A.   Experiences with use of interrupted carmine red and continuous chromium sesquioxide marking of human faeces with reference to calcium, phosphorus, and magnesium. *Gut* 5:274–279, 1964.

48. Rasmussen, H., and Tenenhouse, A.   Thyrocalcitonin, osteoporosis, and osteolysis. *Am. J. Med.* 43:711–726, 1967.

49. Raisz, L. G.   Bone resorption in tissue culture. Factors influenc-

ing the response to parathyroid hormone. *J. Clin. Investigation* 44:103–116, 1965.

50. Goldhaber, P. Heparin enhancement of factors stimulating bone resorption in tissue culture. *Science* 147:407–408, 1965.

51. Golub, L., Glimcher, M. J., and Goldhaber, P. The effect of sodium fluoride on the rates of synthesis and degradation of bone collagen in tissue culture. *Proc. Soc. Exper. Biol. & Med.* 129: 973–977, 1968.

52. Talmage, R. V., and Doty, S. B. Effect of sodium fluoride on parathyroid function in rat as studied by peritoneal lavage. *Gen. & Comp. Endocrinol.* 2:473–479, 1962.

53. Bassett, C. A. L. Biologic significance of piezoelectricity. *Calc. Tiss. Res.* 1:252–272, 1968.

54. Becker, R. O., Bassett, C. A., and Bachman, C. H. Bioelectrical factors controlling bone structure. In Henry Ford Hospital International Symposium. *Bone Biodynamics.* Edited by H. M. Frost. Boston: Little, Brown, 1964. Pp. 209–232.

55. Whedon, G. D. Osteoporosis: atrophy of disuse. In *Bone As a Tissue.* Edited by K. Rodahl, J. T. Nicholson and E. M. Brown. New York: McGraw-Hill, 1960. Pp. 67–82.

56. Burkhart, J. M., and Jowsey, J. Parathyroid and thyroid hormones in development of immobilization osteoporosis. *Endocrinology* 81:1053–1062, 1967.

57. Heaney, R. P. Unpublished data, 1966.

57a. Landry, M., and Fleisch, H. Influence of immobilisation on bone formation as evaluated by osseous incorporation of tetracyclines. *J. Bone & Joint Surg.* 46B:764–771, 1964.

58. Riggs, B. L., Jowsey, J., and Kelly, P. J. Quantitative microradiographic study of bone remodeling in Cushing's syndrome. *Metabolism* 15:773–780, 1966.

59. Harris, W. H. Unpublished data, 1968.

60. Smith, R. W., Jr., and Walker, R. R. Femoral expansion in aging women: implications for osteoporosis and fractures. *Science* 145:156, 1964.

61. Atkinson, P. J., and Weatherell, J. A. Variation in density of femoral diaphysis with age. *J. Bone & Joint Surg.* 49B:781–788, 1967.

62. Urist, M. R. Accelerated aging and premature death of bone cells in osteoporosis. In *Dynamic Studies of Metabolic Bone Disease.* Edited by O. H. Pearson and G. F. Joplin. Philadelphia: Davis, 1964. Pp. 127–160.

63. Sedlin, E. D., Frost, H. M., and Villanueva, A. R. Age changes in resorption in human rib cortex. *J. Gerontol.* 18:345–349, 1963.

64. Newton-John, H. F., and Morgan, D. B. Osteoporosis: disease or senescence? *Lancet* 1:643, 1968.

65. Bell, G. H., Dunbar, O., and Beck, J. S. Variations in strength of vertebrae with age and their relation to osteoporosis. *Calc. Tiss. Res.* 1:75–86, 1967.

References

66. Potts, J. T., Jr., Niall, H. D., Keutmann, H. T., Brewer, H. B., Jr., and Deftos, L. J. Amino acid sequence of porcine thyrocalcitonin. *Proc. Nat. Acad. Sc.* 59:1321–1328, 1968.
67. Foster, G. V. Calcitonin (thyrocalcitonin). *New Eng. J. Med.* 279:349–360, 1968.
68. Pechet, M. M., et al. Symposium on thyrocalcitonin. *Am. J. Med.* 43:645–726, 1967.
68a. *Parathyroid Hormone and Thyrocalcitonin (Calcitonin): Proceedings of the Third Parathyroid Conference: Montreal, Canada, October 16–20, 1967.* Edited by R. V. Talmage and L. F. Bélanger (coeditor, I. Clark). International Congress Series. No. 159. Amsterdam-C., Netherlands: Excerpta Medica, 1968.
69. Walker, D. G. Counteraction to parathyroid therapy in osteopetrotic mice as revealed in plasma calcium level and ability to incorporate ^{3}H-proline into bone. *Endocrinology* 79:836–842, 1966.
70. Johnston, C. C., et al. Osteopetrosis: clinical, genetic, metabolic, and morphologic study of dominately inherited, benign form. *Medicine* 47:149–167, 1968.
71. White, E., and Ahmann, T. M. Calcitonin activity in hereditary osteopetrosis. *J. Clin. Investigation* 44:1111, 1965.
72. Melvin, K. E. W., and Tashjian, A. H., Jr. Syndrome of excessive thyrocalcitonin produced by medullary carcinoma of thyroid. *Proc. Nat. Acad. Sc.* 59:1216–1222, 1968.
73. Tashjian, A. H., Jr., and Munson, P. L. Antibodies to porcine thyrocalcitonin: effects on hypocalcemic activity of calf, rat, and monkey thyroid extracts. *Endocrinology* 77:520–528, 1965.
74. Wells, H., and Lloyd, W. Inhibition of hypocalcemic action of thyrocalcitonin by theophylline and isoproterenol. *Endocrinology* 82:468–474, 1968.
74a. Galante, L., et al. Thyroid and parathyroid origin of calcitonin in man. *Lancet* 2:537–539, 1968.
75. Krane, S. M., Brownell, G. L., Stanbury, J. B., and Corrigan, H. Effect of thyroid disease on calcium metabolism in man. *J. Clin. Investigation* 35:874–887, 1956.
76. Adams, P., and Jowsey, J. Effect of calcium on cortisone-induced osteoporosis: preliminary communication. *Endocrinology* 81:152–154, 1967.
77. Aub, J. C., Albright, F., Bauer, W., and Rossmeisl, E. Studies of calcium and phosphorus metabolism. VI. In hypoparathyroidism and chronic steatorrhea with tetany with special consideration of therapeutic effect of thyroid. *J. Clin. Investigation* 11:211–234, 1932.
78. Harris, W. H., and Heaney, R. P. Effect of growth hormone on skeletal mass in adult dogs. *Nature* (London) 223:403–404, 1969.
79. Frantz, A. G., and Rabkin, M. T. Effects of estrogen and sex difference on secretion of human growth hormone. *J. Clin. Endocrinol. & Metab.* 25:1470–1480, 1965.

References

80. Smith, R. W., Jr. Dietary and hormonal factors in bone loss. *Federation Proc.* 26:1737–1746, 1967.
81. Lafferty, F. W. Discussion of Eisenberg. Effects of corticoids on bone. In *Dynamic Studies of Metabolic Bone Disease*. Edited by O. H. Pearson and G. F. Joplin. Philadelphia: Davis, 1964. P. 124.
82. Pratt, C. W. M. Effects of growth hormone on cellular activities in skeletal tissues of hypophysectomized rat. *Résumé des Communications: Les Tissus Calcifiés*. Fifth Symposium Européen, Bordeaux, France, April 5–8, 1967. P. 39.
83. Heaney, R. P. Radiocalcium metabolism in disuse osteoporosis in man. *Am. J. Med.* 33:188–200, 1962.
83a. Riggs, B. L., Jowsey, J., Kelly, P. J., Jones, J. D., and Maher, F. T. Effect of sex hormones on bone in primary osteoporosis. *J. Clin. Investigation* 48:1065–1072, 1969.
84. Lindquist, B., Budy, A. M., McLean, F. C., and Howard, J. L. Skeletal metabolism in estrogen-treated rats studied by means of Ca⁴⁵. *Endocrinology* 66:100–111, 1960.
85. Lafferty, F. W., Spencer, G. E., Jr., and Pearson, O. H. Effects of androgens, estrogens and high calcium intakes on bone formation and resorption in osteoporosis. *Am. J. Med.* 36:514–528, 1964.
86. Schwartz, E., Panariello, V. A., and Saeli, J. Radioactive calcium kinetics during high calcium intake in osteoporosis. *J. Clin. Investigation* 44:1547–1560, 1965.
87. Henneman, P. H., and Wallach, S. Review of prolonged use of estrogens and androgens in postmenopausal and senile osteoporosis. *Arch. Int. Med.* 100:715–723, 1957.
88. Davis, M. E., Strandjord, N. M., and Lanzl, L. H. Estrogens and aging process: detection, prevention, and retardation of osteoporosis. *J.A.M.A.* 196:219–224, 1966.
88a. Meema, H. E. and Meema, S. Prevention of postmenopausal osteoporosis by hormone treatment of menopause. *Canad. M. A. J.* 99:248–251, 1968.
89. Storey, E. Effect of continuous administration of cortisone and its withdrawal on bone. *Australia & New Zealand J. Surg.* 27: 19–30, 1957.
90. *Idem.* Bone changes associated with cortisone administration in rat: effect of variations in dietary calcium and phosphorus. *Brit. J. Exper. Path.* 41:207–213, 1960.
91. Follis, R. H., Jr. Effect of cortisone on growing bones of rat. *Proc. Soc. Exper. Biol. & Med.* 76:722–724, 1951.
92. Sissons, H. A., and Hadfield, G. J. Influence of cortisone on structure and growth of bone. *J. Anat.* 89:69–78, 1955.
93. Stanisavljevic, S., Roth, H., Villanueva, A. R., and Frost, H. M. Effect of adrenal corticoids on lamellar bone formation rate in rat diaphysis. *Henry Ford Hosp. M. Bull.* 10:179–184, 1962.
94. Eisenberg, E., and Gordan, G. Skeletal dynamics in man mea-

References

sured by nonradioactive strontium. *J. Clin. Investigation* 40: 1809–1825, 1961.

95. Haymovitz, A., and Horwith, M. Miscible calcium pool in metabolic bone disease—in particular, acromegaly. *J. Clin. Endocrinol. & Metab.* 24:4–14, 1964.

96. Gordan, G. S., and Eisenberg, E. Effect of oestrogens, androgens and corticoids on skeletal kinetics in man. *Proc. Roy. Soc. Med.* 56:1027–1029, 1963.

97. Heaney, R. P., Walch, J. J., Steffes, P., and Skillman, T. G. Periarticular bone remodeling in rheumatoid arthritis. In *Proceedings of the 6th European Symposium on Calcified Tissues: Held in Lund, Sweden, Aug. 21–24, 1968. Calc. Tiss. Res.* 2 (Suppl. 1):33–33B, 1968.

98. Fleisch, H., Maerki, J., and Russell, R. G. G. Effect of pyrophosphate on dissolution of hydroxyapatite and its possible importance in calcium homeostasis. *Proc. Soc. Exper. Biol. & Med.* 22:317–320, 1966.

99. Avioli, L. V., McDonald, J. E., Henneman, P. H., and Lee, S. W. Relationship of parathyroid activity to pyrophosphate excretion. *J. Clin. Investigation* 45:1093–1102, 1966.

100. Posen, S. Alkaline phosphatase. *Ann. Int. Med.* 67:183–203, 1967.

101. Woods, C. G. Histological studies in osteomalacia. *J. Bone & Joint Surg.* 48B:188, 1966.

102. Engfeldt, B., Zetterstrom, R., and Winberg, J. Primary vitamin D-resistant rickets. III. Biophysical studies of skeletal tissue. *J. Bone & Joint Surg.* 38A:1323–1327, 1956.

103. Steendijk, R., Jowsey, J., van den Hooff, A., and Nielsen, H. K. L. Microradiographic and histological studies in vitamin D-resistant rickets. In *L'Ostéomalacie*. Edited by D. J. Hioco. Paris: Masson, 1967. Pp. 127–135.

104. Bohr, H. H. Microradiographic studies in osteomalacia. In *L'Ostéomalacie*. Edited by D. J. Hioco. Paris: Masson, 1967. Pp. 117–125.

105. Joplin, G. F., Robinson, C. J., Melvin, K. E. W., Thompson, G. R., and Fraser, R. Results of tracer studies in osteomalacia. In *L'Ostéomalacie*. Edited by D. J. Hioco. Paris: Masson, 1967. Pp. 249–256.

106. Nagant de Deuxchaisnes, C., and Krane, S. M. Treatment of adult phosphate diabetes and Fanconi syndrome with neutral sodium phosphate. *Am. J. Med.* 43:508–543, 1967.

107. Heaney, R. P. Interpretation of kinetic studies in disorders of mineralization. In *L'Ostéomalacie*. Edited by D. J. Hioco. Paris: Masson, 1967. Pp. 239–247.

108. Haas, H. G., Canary, J. J., Kyle, L. H., Meyer, R. J., and Schaaf, M. Skeletal calcium retention in osteoporosis and in osteomalacia. *J. Clin. Endocrinol. & Metab.* 23:605–614, 1963.

109. Lotz, M., Zisman, E., and Bartter, F. C. Evidence for phos-

phorus depletion syndrome in man. *New Eng. J. Med.* 278:409–415, 1968.

110. Wendeberg, B. Mineral metabolism of fractures of tibia in man studied with external counting of Sr^{85}. *Acta Orthop. Scandinav.* Supp. 52:1–79, 1961.

110a. Mack, P. B., LaChance, P. A., Vose, G. P., and Vogt, F. B. Bone demineralization of foot and hand of Gemini-Titan IV, V, and VII astronauts during orbital flight. *Am. J. Roentgenol.* 100:503–511, 1967.

110b. Mack, P. B., and LaChance, P. A. Effects of recumbency and space flight on bone density. *Am. J. Clin. Nutrition* 20:1194–1205, 1967.

111. Lachmann, E., and Whelan, M. Roentgen diagnosis of osteoporosis and its limitations. *Radiology* 26:165–177, 1936.

112. Lachmann, E. Osteoporosis: potentialities and limitations of its roentgenologic diagnosis. *Am. J. Roentgenol.* 74:712–715, 1955.

113. Dent, C. E., and Watson, L. Osteoporosis. *Postgrad. M. J.* Supp., pp. 3–28, October, 1966.

114. Urist, M. R., MacDonald, N. S., Moss, M. J., and Skoog, W. A. Rarefying disease of skeleton: observations dealing with aged and dead bone in patients with osteoporosis. In *Mechanisms of Hard Tissue Destruction.* Edited by R. F. Sognnaes. Washington, D. C.: American Association for the Advancement of Science, 1963. Pp. 385–446.

115. Spencer, H., Menczel, J., and Lewin, I. Metabolic and radioisotope studies in osteoporosis. *Clin. Orthop.* 35:202–219, 1964.

116. Albright, F., Bloomberg, E., and Smith, P. H. Post-menopausal osteoporosis. *Tr. A. Am. Physicians* 55:298–305, 1940.

117. Dymling, J. F. Calcium kinetics in osteopenia and parathyroid disease. *Acta Med. Scandinav.* 175 (Supp. 408) :1–56, 1964.

118. Ray, R. D., Mueller, K. H., Sankaran, B., Mensen, E. D., and Schwartz, T. B. Metabolic diseases of bone: kinetic studies. *M. Clin. North America* 49:241–258, 1965.

119. Fraser, R., Harrison, M., and Ibbertson, K. Rate of calcium turnover in bone. *Quart. J. Med.* 24:85–111, 1960.

120. Villanueva, A. R., et al. Cortical bone dynamics measured by means of tetracycline labeling in 21 cases of osteoporosis. *J. Lab. & Clin. Med.* 68:599–616, 1966.

121. Dallas, I., and Nordin, B. E. C. Relation between calcium intake and roentgenologic osteoporosis. *Am. J. Clin. Nutrition* 11:263–269, 1962.

122. Heaney, R. P. Unified concept of osteoporosis. *Am. J. Med.* 39:877–880, 1965.

123. Young, M. M., and Nordin, B. E. C. Effects of natural and artificial menopause on plasma and urinary calcium and phosphorus. *Lancet* 2:118–120, 1967.

124. Kelly, P. J., Jowsey, J., Riggs, B. L., and Elveback, L. R. Rela-

tionship between serum phosphate concentration and bone resorption in osteoporosis. *J. Lab. & Clin. Med.* 29:110–115, 1967.

125. Shambaugh, G. E., Jr., and Petrovic, A. Effects of sodium fluoride on bone: application to otosclerosis and other decalcifying bone diseases. *J.A.M.A.* 204:969–973, 1968.

126. Nordin, B. E. C. Calcium balance and calcium requirement in spinal osteoporosis. *Am. J. Clin. Nutrition* 10:384–390, 1962.

127. Jowsey, J. Bone in parathyroid disorders in man. In International Congress Series. No. 159. *Parathyroid Hormone and Thyrocalcitonin (Calcitonin): Proceedings of the third Parathyroid Conference: Montreal, Canada, October 16–20, 1967.* Edited by R. V. Talmage and L. F. Bélanger (coeditor: I. Clark). Amsterdam C, Netherlands: Excerpta Medica, 1968. Pp. 137–151.

128. Takahashi, H., Frost, H. M., and Kuhn, T. Bone tissue and cell dynamics determined by tetracycline labeling in case of pseudohypoparathyroidism (and in patient's mother). *Clin. Orthop.* 49: 163–168, 1966.

129. Baylink, D., Morey, E., and Rich, C. Effect of calcitonin on the rates of bone formation and resorption in the rat. *Endocrinology* 84:261–269, 1969.

INDEX

Adrenocortical steroids, 51–53
Age, effects of, 22, 23–24, 29, 39–41, 62–70
Albright, Fuller, hypothesis of, 64
Anabolic agents. *See* Hormones, gonadal
Aubert and Milhaud formulation. *See* Heaney and Whedon formulation

Bauer-Carlsson-Lindquist formula, 14, 15, 18, 30
Bone mass decreased in osteoporosis, 66
Bone mineral metabolism and tracer technics, 13
Bone resorption. *See* Resorption process

"Calcification front," 4–5
Calcitonin, 31, 32, 36, 43
Calcium absorption from diet, 50
Calcium balance, 49
  in hyperparathyroidism, 74
  in hypothyroidism, 47
  measurements, 30
  in osteoporosis, 70–71, 72
Calcium compartments, 18–19
Calcium deficiency
  and osteomalacia, 58
  and osteoporosis, 68
Calcium glycerophosphate, 72
Calcium intake, changes in, 38
Calcium-kinetic methods of measuring skeletal renewal, 13–21, 36, 57
Calcium levels and calcitonin, 44
Calcium-phosphate deposits, 6

Calcium pool, 15
Calcium return, 37
Calcium tracer (s), 14, 18, 21
  studies in osteoporosis, 64, 65, 66
  uptake by bone, 16
Calcium, values for, 20–21
Cancellous bone, 27–28
Carbonate, bone, 5–6
Carcinoma, parathyroid, and calcitonin, 45, 46
Collagen, 4, 34
Corticosteroids. *See* Adrenocortical steroids
Crystal, hydroxyapatite, 6–7
Cushing's syndrome, 37, 52–53

Electrical fields, hypothesis of, 33–34
Enzymatic deficiency, 59
Enzymes, 9
Exchange, long-term, 16–17, 19

Fanconi syndrome, 56
Females, postmenopausal, 48, 50–51, 63–64, 68, 69, 71
Fluid, extracellular, 4, 6, 32
Fluoride
  and osteoporosis, 72
  and parathyroid hormone, 32
Fracture and osteoporosis, 62, 63

Growth hormone, 47–49, 51, 68

Haversian systems. *See* Osteons
Heaney and Whedon formulation, 14–15
Height and loss of skeletal mass, 40

87

Index

Heparin, 70
and parathyroid hormone, 32
Homeostasis, calcium, 10, 31, 66, 69, 72
Hormones
calcitonin, 31, 32, 36, 43
gonadal, and androgens, 49
estrogens, 48, 49, 50–51, 70
role in skeletal renewal, 49–51
synthetic steroids, 49
therapy for osteoporosis, 70–72
growth, 47–49, 51, 68
parathyroid (PTH), 9, 31–36, 73, 75
and calcitonin, 43–44
in osteoporosis, 69–70
tissue response to, 33
thyroid, role in skeletal renewal, 46–47
Hydroxyapatite, crystal, 6–7
Hydroxyproline, 28, 45, 47, 49, 75
Hypercalcemia, 73, 75
Hyperparathyroidism, 36, 44, 56, 73, 75
Hyperthyroidism, 56
and release of calcium from bone, 46–47
Hypocalcemia, 45, 48, 68
Hypoparathyroidism, 36, 56
Hypophosphatasia, 56, 59
Hypophosphatemia, 56, 59
Hypothyroidism, bone effects, 47

Intoxication, bone, 56, 59

Joints, inflamed, and osteoporosis, 62

Lamellae, interstitial, 2

Matrix
components of, 4–5
mineralization, 4, 5, 8, 14, 15, 16, 49
in osteomalacia, 55
Mechanical forces, and bone formation, 34–35
Menopause and loss of skeletal mass, 39

Mesenchyme, bone
functional states of, 3
and remodeling, 2
response to mechanical stimuli, 34–35
Microradiography as measurement, 22
Microscopical studies, problems of, 27–28
Mineralization. *See under* Matrix
Morphometric methods of measuring skeletal renewal, 22–28
Morphometric studies in osteoporosis, 67

Nucleating configuration, 5

Orthophosphate and pyrophosphate, 7
Osteoblast activity in osteoporosis, 64, 66, 68
Osteoblasts, 1, 3
and nucleation, 7–8
Osteoclasts, 3, 9, 31, 32
and parathyroid hormone, 33
Osteocyte, 3
functions of, 10–11
Osteocytic osteolysis, 33
Osteoid borders, 8, 55, 56
Osteomalacia, 24, 55–59
distinguished from osteoporosis, 58
Osteons, 1
number of, and changes with age, 40–41
Osteopetrosis, 44, 45
Osteoporosis
corticosteroid, 60–61
in Cushing's syndrome, 53, 60
defined, 60
from disuse, 33, 35, 37, 46, 69
gonadal hormones in, 50
high-turnover, 61
and hyperthyroid state, 47
local, 61–62
postmenopausal, 45, 46, 62–70, 74
senile, 45, 46, 62–70
space flight, 62

DATE DUE

DEMCO, INC. 38-2931